W9-ANX-075

Outsmarting the Female Fat Cell—After Pregnancy

ALSO BY DEBRA WATERHOUSE, M.P.H., R.D.

Outsmarting Female Food Cravings:
From Chocolate to Cheese—How to Master the Art of Self-Indulgence Without Overindulgence

Outsmarting the Mother–Daughter Food Trap:
How to Free Yourself from Dieting—and Pass On a Healthier Legacy to Your Daughter

Outsmarting Female Fatigue:
Eight Energizing Strategies for Lifelong Vitality

Outsmarting the Midlife Fat Cell:
Winning Weight Control Strategies for Women over 35 to Stay Fit Through Menopause

Outsmarting the Female Fat Cell:
The First Weight-Control Program Designed Specifically for Women

Outsmarting the Female Fat Cell—After Pregnancy

Every Woman's Guide to Shaping Up, Slimming Down, and Staying Sane After the Baby

Debra Waterhouse, M.P.H., R.D.

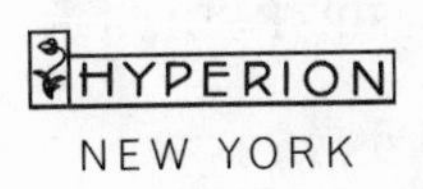

NEW YORK

Copyright © 2002 Debra Waterhouse, M.P.H., R.D.

All rights reserved. No part of this book may be used or reproduced in any manner whatsoever without the written permission of the Publisher. Printed in the United States of America. For information address: Hyperion, 77 W. 66th Street, New York, New York 10023-6298.

Library of Congress Cataloging-in-Publication Data

Waterhouse, Debra.

Outsmarting the female fat cell—after pregnancy : every woman's guide to shaping up, slimming down, and staying sane after the baby / by Debra Waterhouse.—1st ed.

p. cm.

Includes bibliographical references and index.

ISBN 0-7868-6537-7

1. Postnatal care—Popular works. 2. Weight loss—Popular works. 3. Puerperium—Nutritional aspects—Popular works. 4. Exercise for women—Popular works. 5. Physical fitness for women—Popular works. I. Title.

RG801 .W38 2002
618.6—dc21

2001024860

FIRST EDITION

0 9 8 7 6 5 4 3 2 1

To my

TYLER

for
a pregnancy to cherish,
a birth to remember,
and
a life to anticipate with wonder, joy, and excitement

The recommendations in this book are not intended for pregnant women, women with chronic illnesses, or to replace or conflict with advice given to you by your physician or other health professional. All matters regarding your health require medical supervision. Consult your physician before adopting the suggestions in this book. The author and publisher disclaim any liability arising directly or indirectly from the use of this book.

Except for those who have given permission to appear in this book, all names and characteristics of persons have been changed. In some cases, composite accounts have been created based on the author's professional experience.

Acknowledgments

After writing five other books, I thought this one would be a breeze. How difficult could it be to write a book with a new baby? I'd be cooped up at home and not doing much anyway. How hard could it be to find the time to be creative and productive? He'd be sleeping the day away or sitting beside me quietly while I typed away.

Was I in for the surprise of my life! This book was by far the most challenging. Finding the time to get into my creative thoughts was next to impossible; he never sat quietly for more than five minutes and never slept for more than an hour at a time. Without the experience of having a baby, I couldn't have written this book—and with the experience of having a baby in my life, I almost never did.

If it wasn't for the unconditional support of family, friends, sitters, an empathetic editor, and a saint of a sister, I think Tyler would be in the first grade by the time I turned in my manuscript. My sister, Lori, as always, deserves my deepest thanks for not only being my seasoned reviewer but also my resident postpartum expert. Having gone through pregnancy and postbaby weight loss three times, she eagerly read through my drafts with a keen eye and the wisdom of experience.

My incredible editor, Leslie Wells, was forever patient, encouraging, and validating. Her repeated (and cherished) comment, "How I wish I had this book after my son was born! It would have made all the difference in the world," kept me going during the most difficult times. And another amazing woman, Carleen Driscoll, was also instrumental in keeping me going when I didn't think I could. She was my research assistant, computer expert, and child-care provider all rolled into one—and saved my life many times over. Without her, I'm convinced I could never have done it.

I could also never have written this book without Sandra Dijkstra, and my publisher, Hyperion. Sandy Dijkstra and her staff have been behind me, my ideas, and my writing for over a decade. And Bob Miller and his staff have shown unwavering support for my work and have remained my one and only publisher.

I would also like to extend my deepest appreciation to my husband, Paul, for putting up with me staying up all night and staying in all weekend. To my mom and dad, Alina and Ray Waterhouse, and my mother-in-law, Laura Manca, for knowing when to call to check in, and for knowing when not to call to give me my needed writing space. To my friend Stephanie Goulding for reading my manuscript and providing a welcomed distraction to writing and motherhood—her upcoming wedding. And to my female comrades, Dee Tivenan, Michelle Hawkins, Joyce Filatreau, Mary Pat Cedarleaf, Denise Quackenbush, Jeannette Stansbury, Karen McElhatton, Laura Euphrat, and Chrisi Brown, for simply being there.

And lastly, I would like to acknowledge myself. Perhaps a bit self-serving, but nonetheless, well deserved. I am in awe of the fact that I was not only able to complete this book during the demanding first year of my son's life, but to also deliver this manuscript on time and still enjoy every minute of motherhood with my beautiful Tyler. I think some Dom Perignon is in order. Care to join me?

Contents

Introduction

The "Fat Cell Lady" Has to Outsmart Her Own

That's me—the Fat Cell Lady—a nickname I wouldn't necessarily choose for myself, but after writing four books on the subject of female fat cells, I'm no longer surprised when someone introduces me as the "Fat Cell Lady" or inquires about my own fat-cell experiences. Since I had my first child, however, it seems as if just about everyone wants to know what happened to the Fat Cell Lady's fat cells during the nine weight-gaining months of pregnancy.

They had the biggest celebration of their life—that's what happened. All thirty billion of them banned together and rejoiced, "Thank God, she's finally pregnant! For years, she's outsmarted us with her eating and exercise strategies. Now, it's our turn to outsmart her, and she can't do a thing about it." My fat cells took full advantage of their new mother-to-be status by growing, storing, and expanding to their hearts' content. And to be quite honest with you, even though I write books, give seminars, and counsel women on the strong, smart, and stubborn nature of female fat cells, I never truly experienced how powerful they could be until I became pregnant—and never fully realized how ingenious and nonnegotiable they really were until I had to work on outsmarting my own postpartum fat cells.

Thinking back, I remember feeling my fat cells starting to expand before the idea that I could possibly be pregnant even crossed my mind. As my clothes were getting a bit tighter in the waist, I quickly concluded that it must be the next stage of perimenopause kicking in. After years of no birth control and no pregnancy, my husband and I were beginning to resolve ourselves to a life without kids. But then, thankfully, it happened, and my fat cells were the first to know, eager to let me in on their little secret.

Having worked with pregnant and postpartum women for over twenty years, I knew what to do and how to do it. I'd been telling my clients to let their fat cells and hormones do what they needed to do for a healthy pregnancy, and not worry about weight loss until well after delivery. I'd been encouraging them to take care of themselves with food and fitness, and let their bodies gain a healthy amount of weight that was right for them. I'd been supporting them through the painfully slow and arduous weight loss in the postpartum months—helping them to embrace the changes in their bodies and avoid the temptation to diet. But all of my knowledge and skills in helping others still didn't fully prepare me to help myself. First I had to come to terms with pregnant fat cells that never stopped to rest. Then I had to deal with stubborn postpartum fat cells that didn't want to budge.

It wasn't always easy. The first few months of pregnancy were particularly challenging as my body was producing fat without looking pregnant—and I was feeling fat without feeling pregnant. At about twelve weeks into my pregnancy, I remember my husband putting his arms around my waist at a party and commenting, "Wow! You have love handles. I've never felt this much fat on your hips before." When he saw the look on my face, he immediately realized his blunder and continued, "And I like it. I really do. I like you with hips, and I like your bigger boobs, too." Too late, his fat-confirming words were already spoken.

Firmly removing his hand from my waist, I marched directly into the bathroom, yanked up my dress, and analyzed my hips from every possible angle. He wasn't lying and neither was the mirror. Despite my purposeful choice of a slimming, black outfit with ample stretch—the love handles reflected back at me, and I knew I had to get a handle on them. As an impatient line formed outside of the bathroom, I stood there in front of the mirror doing some self-talk, telling myself that the hips are the first place that fat is laid on in quantity for the growing baby and that these love handles were the beautiful product of lovemaking and conceiving. I also tried to divert my attention upward to my growing breasts. They were the biggest they'd ever been in my life. But the truth was that my first B cup was nothing to write home about, and much to my dismay, they stopped growing after the twelfth week. The one enlargement I was seriously looking forward to had abandoned me.

And so did some of my friends. That very same night, one came up to congratulate me, saying, "Oh, you're definitely having a girl because if you were having a boy, you'd be beautiful and glowing by now." First love handles, and now this! My fat cells were growing—but I wasn't glowing. On the verge of tears from raging hormones and heightened sensitivity, I felt pasty and pudgy for the rest of the night. (By the way, as it turned out, this so-called friend was wrong. I did have a boy—a beautiful, healthy, heart-melting boy—and in my opinion, I did glow.)

You may be thinking, "the nerve of that woman" to basically tell me that I was an unattractive, unglowing pregnant woman. But this was only one of the many less-than-complimentary appearance and weight-related comments I received throughout my pregnancy. Although most friends, relatives, and colleagues were extremely happy for my upcoming motherhood, some seemed even happier about my anticipated weight struggles.

- "Now you'll finally know what it's like to have to worry about your weight."
- "I can't wait to watch your flat stomach get fat, flabby, and round."
- "I hope you get a lot of stretch marks and varicose veins."
- "Your body will never be the same, you know; I wonder how you'll handle it."
- "I wonder if you'll bounce back; you're not a spring chicken anymore, you know."

Yes, I knew. I was forty, not twenty. My hormones, body, and fat cells had already been changing due to perimenopause, and my skin, muscles, and metabolism were starting to change due to the aging process. Would I bounce back? I am a woman, not a ball (even though I was starting to resemble one), so I didn't know if it was even possible to "bounce back." And although some of these comments caused brief moments of self-doubt, I vowed not to let myself be one of the 72 percent of women who wasted precious time and energy fearing future weight struggles in the postpartum months. The health of my developing baby was more important than potential stretch marks, weight struggles, and a body that wouldn't bounce back. All I could do was follow my own advice: feed my body well, keep it active, keep my fingers crossed, and let nature take its course.

As my fat cells continued to take their course by expanding to 125 percent of their original size, the most commonly asked question was not, "When are you due?" or "Do you know what you're having?"; it was "How much weight have you gained?" I guess people assumed that my profession allowed such personal questions, and most were not satisfied with my answer, which was always, "I don't know."

I honestly didn't know. I had no idea what my prepregnancy weight was because I never got on the scale. I hold the very strong belief that the bathroom scale only serves to zap our self-esteem. It's a mechanical device that determines whether we leave the house with a smile or a frown—and nothing made of metal should have that kind of power over our happiness. During pregnancy, however, the scale is deemed necessary to make sure that we're gaining enough weight for the health of our babies.

I don't know about you, but I knew I was gaining enough weight. My fat cells were reminding me every day. I didn't need a scale to tell me that it was time to live in my sweatpants, wear my husband's shirts, or buy bigger maternity clothes. My body accurately informed me that I wasn't gaining too little weight, and if I was gaining too much weight—then so be it. I wasn't excessively overindulging, I wasn't eating ice cream sundaes every day, and I wasn't using pregnancy as an excuse to eat nonstop morning, noon, and night. Instead, I ate when I was hungry (which was often), ate what my body wanted (which was huge amounts of yogurt, cheese, and a surprising amount of sugar), and let my body gain the amount of weight it needed to gain for a healthy pregnancy.

But exactly how much weight did I gain? You probably want to know the answer to that question, and my answer is still, "I don't know." But if I were to guess based on weigh-ins at my prenatal visits, I'd say somewhere between thirty-five and forty pounds by the time I went into labor three weeks early.

People tell me I was lucky to "go early," especially with a first child, but I wasn't ready. I wasn't ready with his room or my hospital bag. I wasn't ready to stop being pregnant. I'm one of those women who loved being pregnant and loved my swollen belly, and I wanted to enjoy both during those last few weeks. But he couldn't wait. He wanted out, and he wanted out quick. Everyone told me that the first child takes hours, possibly days, but my contractions were two minutes apart within an hour and by the time I made it to the hospital, I was almost fully dilated and in transition. Which is not to say I had an easy labor. He decided to hang out for a while behind my pelvic bone and took his time as he tore (literally) into the world.

Although childbirth classes try to prepare you for labor and delivery, nothing can really prepare you for your own unique experience. All of my classes, reading, and talking to women about their labor-room stories didn't do justice to the magnitude of pain I experienced while pushing or the unsurpassed pleasure I felt while gazing at his cone-shaped head for the very first time. But what surprised me the most was that I had virtually no preparation for what happened after delivery—the cramping, the pain, the bleeding, the exhaustion, and the lengthy recovery. I had no idea that I would look seven-months pregnant for the next few weeks, or that I would have night sweats every hour on the hour, or that I would cry every time my baby cried, or that the breastfeeding latch-on technique, newborn cord care, infant baths, and meconium-filled diaper changes would not be driven by instinct.

I laugh now at my prebaby vision of maternity leave, thinking that I would be relaxing side-by-side with my infant, reading novels, taking naps, strolling in the park, and meeting friends for lunch. In the weeks following delivery, I could barely think, never mind do anything. I was lucky if I remembered to brush my teeth by noon, and if I managed to bathe both my baby and myself in the same day, it was a monumental accomplishment.

What I did read about the weeks following delivery told me that I'd be up and walking by the second day (unless I had a C-section), doing modified sit-ups by the second week, fully recovered by the fourth, having sex again by the sixth, and fitting back into my prepregnancy clothes by the eighth. The reality was that I could barely get out of bed on the second day, doing nothing but breastfeeding and changing diapers at the second week, still bleeding at the fourth, cringing at the thought of sex at the sixth, and still wearing maternity stretch pants at the eighth. How was I supposed to walk when I could barely stand? How was I supposed to do sit-ups when it still hurt to sit down? How was I supposed to wear my favorite pants when I couldn't get them up beyond my thighs?

Was there something wrong with me or was there something the matter with the books and postpartum educational materials? After talking to other new moms, I quickly concluded that nothing was wrong with me; the information out there was flawed, painting an unrealistic picture of the postpartum months. One book I read said that you should be able to slip into your Levi's with ease at six weeks; another promised that you could weigh less at six months than before you got pregnant; another said that breastfeeding was a surefire way to melt away the fat and "get your body back" within two months; and yet another declared that you should be running by the second month, and running marathons by the sixth.

No wonder women feel as if they are failing the postpartum body test, and struggling to lose after-the-baby pounds—their expectations were grossly misguided in the first place. If women were informed upfront that it would take nine months to a year or more to lose the twenty pounds of fat they gained in pregnancy, and that the last five to ten pounds would be the most stubborn despite their efforts to exercise, eat healthy, and breastfeed—perhaps they wouldn't feel as frustrated with themselves or as confused about their uncooperative fat cells.

Are you frustrated and confused? According to a study published in the journal *Birth,* new mothers were more confused about how to care for their own bodies than how to care for their babies. They had more questions about what to eat, when to eat, how much to eat, when to exercise, how much to exercise, and what to do about fatigue, sleeplessness, hair loss, and depression—than about how to feed, bathe, and change their babies. But who can we turn to for answers? The medical community provides thorough prenatal care, but from the minute you leave the hospital, postnatal care is almost nonexistent. Your obstetrician checks you at six weeks for recovery below the belt, and your only chance to ask your pressing questions is while you're immobilized in stirrups. Then most of us don't see our doctors again for another year. In the interim, I suppose postnatal classes would be great, but what new mother has the time, energy, and resources to go? A number of organizations have tried offering classes, but even with free child care, the rooms were almost always empty.

As we were discussing the lack of attention on postpartum care and weight loss, one of my clients added, "And everyone's attention is focused on my baby's weight gain, not on my weight loss. Everyone wants to know how my daughter is doing with breastfeeding and how much weight she's gained, but no one asks me how I'm doing with eating and weight loss. Except for my mother-in-law, that is. She's convinced that I'm going to 'let myself go' and become an overweight wife and mother, and she's constantly reminding me how she left the hospital wearing her size six honeymoon outfit. I want to prove her wrong, but I need help."

This book will give you all the help you need by bringing the focus back to you, answering your questions honestly, and dispelling the postbaby body myths with the latest research. It may not be exactly what you *want* to hear—but it's precisely what you *need* to hear to set the record straight about postpartum weight.

- **You will *not* leave the hospital wearing your favorite prepregnancy outfit—** but you know that already since you left in the same maternity clothes you arrived in. If you happen to know someone who did, she's an anomaly who should be featured in *Ripley's Believe It or Not.*

- **You will *not* "get your body back" within two months—** unless you're twenty years old and genetically blessed with a fast metabolism and a lean figure. And how could you "get your body back," anyway? It was never gone. It's been right there with you every step of the way, performing the miracle of life.

- **You will *not* weigh less than before you were pregnant—** unless you were overweight before and viewed pregnancy and the postpartum months as an opportunity to take care of yourself through food and fitness. Then you'll not only lose all your pregnancy pounds, but you may lose a few extra ones that probably should have been outsmarted years ago. For the rest of us, however, reaching our prepregnancy weight is the most we can hope for, and it's more likely we'll miss the target by a few pounds. The average woman holds on to an extra two to five pounds after the baby.

- **You will *not* be up and running within a few weeks—** unless you had a two-hour labor with no tearing or stitches, and a full-time nanny from day one. Even then, it's doubtful you'll be pounding the pavement. Even if you feel ready to run, walk, or swim, your baby isn't ready to let you out of his or her sight.

- **You will *not* melt away the fat by breastfeeding—** unless you do it exclusively for six months to a year. Most studies have shown little correlation between breastfeeding and weight loss prior to six months, and some have even found that those women who bottle-feed lose more weight. Surprised that the breast isn't always the best for weight loss? But that's no reason to burn your nursing bras and try to get your baby to turn the other cheek; the benefits of lactation for you and your infant are unsurpassed. And you can outsmart your fat cells while breastfeeding. You just have to know how to work with your lactating hormones.

- **You will *not* be wearing your Levi's at six weeks—** unless you go out and buy new Levi's. The six-week recovery myth has done as much damage to women's self-esteem as the six-foot, 110-pound modeling industry. How could you expect your body to recover in 42 days after 277 days of pregnancy and a ten-hour (if you're lucky) labor? Even at six months, one in four women still don't feel fully recovered, and 90 percent are still unable to squeeze into their jeans.

I couldn't, and I'm the Fat Cell Lady. My life's work is dedicated to shrinking fat cells. As I write this introduction, it's been about eight months since I had Tyler, and my Levi's are still sitting at the bottom of the drawer. Breastfeeding has caused me to hang on to pregnancy fat, and I'm walking with no desire to run marathons (which has nothing to do with pregnancy; I wouldn't be running marathons, anyway). But on the positive side, I have lost most of the weight, burned away most of the fat, fit into most of my clothes, and I'm having the most fun I've ever had in my life. Right now, "most" is good enough for me, and I want to help make it good enough for you, too.

I may be the Fat Cell Lady, but I'm not any different from you. My postpartum fat loss has been slow and steady. Sometimes stubborn. Sometimes stymied. But always on my body's schedule, not mine. Personally, I would have loved to have been back to my fit and firm self by bathing-suit season, but I wasn't. I would have loved to have worn my favorite backless cocktail dress for that important party, but I couldn't. My body wasn't ready yet, and I wasn't ready to take time away from my little one, Tyler, to spend hours at the gym aerobicizing, body sculpting, and weight training. What if I missed a first smile, a first tooth, a first step, or a first word? And I wasn't about to contemplate some quick weight-loss diet to try to speed up the process. As one of the leaders in the antidieting movement, I knew better. You can't force your postpartum fat cells to release fat. No postpregnancy diet, weight loss drink, fat-burning pill, or metabolism-boosting herb will shrink your fat cells back to their prepregnancy size. In fact, dieting will only cause your fat cells to protect their precious storage of calories. Studies from the United States, Sweden, and elsewhere have found that those women who diet in the postpartum months hold on to *twice* as much fat as those who simply eat moderately and start exercising.

Needless to say, I never dieted, never skipped a meal, never popped a diet pill, and never did hundreds of crunches a day. But I did exercise three days a week (often with Tyler on my back), ate five small meals a day, and outsmarted my fat cells to the best of my ability. And I continue to do so. My waist may be a bit larger, my hips permanently stuck in a slightly wider position, and my breasts smaller than ever, but I'm not overly concerned about it because I know that my body will continue to change on its own schedule.

If you are not yet a new mother, but instead a mother-to-be, please close this book for now. And instead open the cupboard, eat well, take your prenatals, stay active, and don't worry about weight loss until after you've delivered your baby. A surprising number of women are restricting their eating and weight gain during pregnancy, in the hopes that they'll have an easier time losing weight after. One study found that over 30 percent of new mothers admitted to undereating during pregnancy for the sole purpose of weight control. Has our obsession with thinness gone so far as to jeopardize the health of our developing babies?

Although a few studies have found that those women who gain the least amount of weight during pregnancy have the easiest time losing it, all studies have found that those who restrict weight gain increase their chances of premature births, stillbirths, and low-birth-weight infants. And there's no guarantee anyway that a smaller pregnancy weight gain will make you a smaller postpartum woman. Women who gain fifty pounds can lose the weight more quickly than those who gain only twenty-five pounds. There are no "rules" when it comes to successful postpartum weight loss. Your age, prepregnancy weight, pregnancy weight gain, birth weight of your infant, and even the number of pregnancies and multiple births you've had—are *not* determining factors in your weight loss. *How you approach weight loss in the postpartum months is what determines success.*

I've already said that dieting is *not* the approach you want; it only makes your fat cells hold on to their fat for dear life. So, what can you do to outsmart your postpartum fat cells? You can follow the Postpartum Peace Plan—a mother-friendly weight-loss program with the goal to help you realistically make peace with your fat cells, food, fitness, and female body. It includes:

- **A realistic timeline that addresses your unique needs from the first six weeks through the next six years.** Other than the twelve pounds you lost on the delivery table (the quickest weight-loss diet you'll ever go on!), the majority of your weight won't even start to come off until well after the three-month mark. And what you do between three and nine months is the most instrumental in outsmarting your fat cells forever.

- **Realistic eating and exercise strategies designed to work with your new postpartum body and your new, time-consuming postbaby life.** Research from one of the largest studies to date, the Stockholm Pregnancy and Weight Development Study, found that those women who lost the most weight had the most regular and consistent meal schedule. They ate three meals a day plus a snack or two, and never missed a feeding. It wasn't *what* they ate, but *when* they ate that made the difference. I might also add that they never missed an exercise session. They faithfully moved their bodies four hours a week—and it didn't matter what activity they chose.

- **Realistic goals of what your postbaby body can ultimately achieve.** If you expect your body to look exactly like it did before it went through nine months of fat storage, you're setting yourself up for disappointment, depression, and body dissatisfaction. A study from Australia found that unrealistic postpartum weight expectations triggered poor body image and increased the risk of depression. That risk can be greatly reduced when expectations are more in line with biological realities.

As you can tell, I'm a big fan of being realistic. How can you be anything but realistic when your life has just been turned upside down with an infant who needs twenty-four-hour love and care? You know that it would be impossible to keep the schedule you did before you got pregnant, or follow a specific food plan that required hours of preparation, or make it to your noon step-aerobics class every Monday, Wednesday, and Friday. And if this is your second, third, or fourth child, "being realistic" takes on a whole new meaning. With the addition of a toddler who needs a watchful eye, a school-ager who needs a full-time taxi driver, and a teenager who still needs you (but doesn't think she does), you have no choice but to be realistic.

Whatever your life situation, I'll outline the most time-sensitive timeline and the most successful strategies in helping you to shape up and slim down—but after the ups and downs, please understand that your body will be slightly different as a tribute to the remarkable experience of birth. It will be stronger, healthier, sexier, curvier, wiser, more confident, and more accomplished. It will be different *and better*.

When you stop and think about what your body did to create life, deliver it, feed it, and nurture it, you can't help but marvel at its strength, power, pain tolerance, resiliency, and life-giving qualities. It just accomplished the most phenomenal physical feat in the world, putting men's physical capabilities to shame. As you read through these pages, acknowledge the strength of your body, marvel at the miracle of birth, change what you can, accept what you can't, eat well, move your body, laugh often, play with your children, and immerse yourself in the joys of motherhood.

Whether you're holding on to five extra pounds or fifty, I'd like this book to be your real-world resource for postpregnancy life. Not just for information on weight, fat, food, and exercise—but also on setting priorities, caring for yourself, balancing your life, and overcoming the challenges that sometimes come with motherhood: self-doubt, body dissatisfaction, role conflict, ongoing stress, sleepless nights, overwhelming fatigue, hair loss, constipation, urinary problems, and depression. Whether you had your baby a week ago (where did you find the time to even open this book?!), a month ago, a year ago, or five years ago, this book is your complete, step-by-step guide that's breastfeeding-friendly, body image–boosting, fat-burning, metabolism-elevating, muscle-toning, tummy-tightening, sleep-enhancing, sex-stimulating, fatigue-fighting, stress-reducing, mood-enhancing, hair-restoring, and even hemorrhoid-healing and constipation-controlling—all rolled into one. Because I not only want to help you shape up and slim down, I also want to help you save your sanity at the same time. *After all, what good is a fit, toned body if you can't enjoy every waking—and sleeping—moment!*

Chapter One

Those Pesky, Persnickety Postpartum Pounds

An hour after you delivered your baby, you still look nine months pregnant but are too exhilarated and exhausted to notice. A day later, you finally gaze down in amazement at your protruding, squishy stomach, but the sight of your beautiful newborn quickly distracts you. A week later, on your first venture out to the store, someone asks you when the baby is due, and the shocking reality of your postbaby body comes into full focus. A month later, you're still living in your maternity stretch pants and despise them more each day. Three months later, most anything that zips, snaps, or buttons is still in storage, and you decide it's time to wage war against your waistline. Six months later, you're still battling the postbaby bulge and feel like you're losing the war but not the weight. A year later, you're still a full size larger and institute a "no sex" policy, declaring that you're never getting pregnant again. A decade and two more pregnancies later, your oldest child is entering adolescence, and you're too busy coping with their body changes to worry about your own anymore.

If you feel as though you're under a dark cloud of stubborn, postpartum fat cells—let me enlighten you. Of the 350,000 women around the world who delivered a baby today, 95 percent of them will struggle for months and possibly years with postpartum weight loss. Somewhere in the midst of that struggle, half will give up and surrender to their fat cells, becoming overweight mothers for the rest of their lives. The other half will give in to restrictive dieting to combat postbaby fat, becoming starving mothers for the rest of their lives.

Where are you in the fight against postpartum pounds? Are you ready to give up and throw in the towel? Or are you contemplating giving in to starvation and throwing diet pills in your mouth? Before you go to either extreme, keep reading this book. You don't have to be an overweight *or* a starving mother. With the necessary knowledge and skills to permanently outsmart your postpartum fat cells, you can become a body-accepting mother who eats regularly, enjoys food, stays fit, and maintains a comfortable weight. *You can become a mother, partner, and woman who has a healthy, peaceful relationship with food and her body.*

You just need to know the facts about after-the-baby fat. Contrary to what you may have read or been told, losing weight after the baby is no easy feat. It may be the toughest weight loss you'll ever encounter—you just stored twelve to twenty pounds of fat in nine months, and once that fat is residing comfortably in your fat cells, it wants to stay put for as long as possible. Recent research has uncovered just how stubborn postpartum weight loss really is: Six months after the baby, most women are battling at least ten extra pounds, and a year later, less than 25 percent have returned to their prepregnancy weight.

But these statistics probably come as no surprise to you. Whether you had your baby six weeks, six months, or six years ago, you've had firsthand experience with resistant postpartum fat cells. You're living proof that postbaby weight loss is painfully slow and particularly stubborn. Like most of my clients, however, you're probably wondering why you weren't informed of these weight loss realities up front—and why instead you were led to believe that you'd be fully recovered within six weeks, lose most of the weight by eight weeks, and look like you never bore a child at twelve weeks. The answer is: because much of the material available to us is either outdated or outlandish. Your body recently went through 277 days of pregnancy—how could it possibly recover in just 42 days? Your body just completed the most amazing physical transformation of your life, where your waist expanded to fifty inches, your skin stretched by 400 percent, your abdominal muscles pulled apart by 300 percent, your uterus grew ten sizes, your hips widened by half a foot, and your fat cells grew to 125 percent of their original size. How could it bounce back to a nonpregnancy state in just two or three months? It can't—it's a physical impossibility.

Eight months after having my first child, I still hadn't lost all the weight. And my life's work is dedicated to shrinking female fat cells! I personally don't know of any woman who was back to her prepregnant self within eight or twelve weeks. If you do—*show me the mommy!* Unless you're a twenty-year-old aerobics instructor who had a two-hour labor and is genetically blessed with a fast metabolism, your body will take months, not weeks, to fully recover, realign your bones, readjust your muscles, return your skin tone, and release the stored fat from your fat cells.

So, instead of giving up and doing nothing or giving in to a life of restriction and eating nothing, consider a third option: *understanding exactly what's going on in your postbaby body and realistically outsmarting your postpartum fat cells by working with their stubborn nature.* When you arm yourself with knowledge, you'll have all the ammunition you need to shape up, slim down, and shrink your fat cells forever.

BELLIES AND BOTTOMS AND BOOBS . . . OH MY!

Where is your body holding on to the most fat? Which fat cells are ignoring your efforts in weight loss? It may be all thirty billion of them (yes, you have thirty billion fat cells that were thrilled to grow during your pregnancy), or those located primarily in your stomach, hips, buttocks, breasts, and thighs. The number one trouble spot for new mothers is their stomach—the "abominable abdominals," the "troublesome tummy," the "squishy stomach," the "jelly belly"—or any other name you've given it. Next on the list of body grievances come the "hippopotamus hips," the "bulging buttocks," the "thunder thighs," and the "big boobs." The areas of your body that grew the largest during the fat-storing months of pregnancy stay the largest during the fat-resistant months of postpartum recovery.

Before we uncover the truth about your pesky, persnickety postpartum pounds, let's first discuss what happened during your nine fat-storing months of pregnancy. The moment that triumphant sperm successfully penetrated the egg, hormones were released to start preparing your body for a healthy pregnancy. Many different hormones are involved in pregnancy, but estrogen and progesterone are the key players in protecting the fertilized egg, stimulating the growth of your baby, and signaling your fat cells to store fat like never before. Ever since you went through puberty, your fat cells were anxiously awaiting that day of conception. As soon as they got the express message from estrogen that a special delivery was coming in nine months, their purpose in life was called to action. "Bingo! We have a winner! Let's not waste any time; we have an important job to do to keep her and her baby healthy. Ready, set, store!"

Your fat cells were informed of your pregnancy before you were, and started to grow before you missed your first period. And they kept growing for nine months straight without rest, sleep, or coffee breaks. The high estrogen levels of pregnancy ensured their growth by activating the fat storage enzymes. These enzymes work as carriers to transport calories into your fat cells for storage, and the more enzymes you have, the more calories you can store—and the bigger your fat cells can become. When you were pregnant, those enzymes at least doubled in number and strength, and your fat cells became twice as efficient at storing the calories from the ice cream, pickles, doughnuts, chocolate éclairs, cookies, Chinese food, and every other food you ate during your pregnancy. You weren't just eating for two; you were eating for thirty billion—thirty billion fat cells, that is. And they were ecstatic with your new no-holds-barred eating attitude. Even if you didn't use pregnancy as permission to eat anything and everything in sight, your fat cells were still able to scoop up every possible calorie from every possible food. Even if you had the world's worse case of morning sickness, your fat cells were still able to salvage what you could keep down. Whatever your eating situation, your fat cells successfully grew because your fat-storage enzymes doubled in their ability to store.

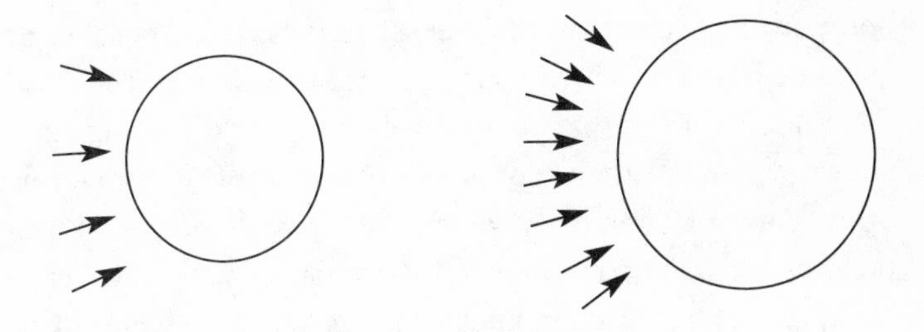

Fat-storing Before Pregnancy   Fat-storing During Pregnancy

The weight you gained during pregnancy was not by chance; it was carefully planned by your fat cells. Nor was it random; it followed a specific blueprint from your female biology. The fat cells of your breasts, hips, abdomen, buttocks, and thighs were the first to be activated because their location played a vital role during your pregnancy. Your breasts needed more fat to prepare for breastfeeding;

your abdomen, hips, and buttocks needed larger fat cells to cushion the growing fetus; and your thighs were just along for the ride, storing extra calories in case you needed them.

Love handles, a pouched belly, jiggling thighs, and swaying breasts—these were the first signs that estrogen and your fat cells were doing their job. Estrogen is more likely to increase the storage of what's called subcutaneous fat, the fat that's located right under your skin. It's what you can see, pinch, grab, and jiggle. It's also the fat that protects the fetus and provides the thirty thousand calories necessary for labor and delivery. If you didn't store all that subcutaneous fat, you wouldn't have had the energy to push nonstop for hours without a bite to eat. And you wouldn't have had any energy left to coo and cuddle your baby immediately after that longest and most intense workout of your life.

In the first twenty weeks of pregnancy, your body instinctively knew to store mostly subcutaneous fat in your breasts and your lower body. In the second twenty weeks, your body purposefully directed more of your calories to your placenta for the growth of your baby. That doesn't mean that your fat cells called it quits midway through your pregnancy—they kept growing, too—but the storage spread to other parts of your body. Once the fat cells of your hips, thighs, breasts, and abdomen were filled to capacity, the fat cells of your back, arms, cheeks, chin, knees, fingers, and toes were thrilled to be called upon to help out with your weight gain. So after delivery, even though women are most dissatisfied with their abdomen and thighs, they are also less than pleased with their chipmunk cheeks, double chins, chubby ringless fingers, and back fat that protrudes up over their bra straps.

And the body dissatisfaction intensifies with each week after delivery. For the first six weeks, women are slightly dissatisfied with their postpartum bodies, but by twelve weeks they are downright frustrated, and at twenty-four weeks they have the phone numbers handy for the diet doctor and the liposuction surgeon. They are at war with their bodies without really knowing the "enemy."

Are you? Are you trying to battle the postbaby bulge without knowing the facts about your stubborn postpartum fat cells? Well, *the harder you try to fight them, the stronger they'll become.* As you'll soon find out, dieting will only result in more active fat cells that are more efficient at storage. Your fat cells will conquer any pill, drink, herb, food, or plan you use as your diet weapon. Unfortunately, they will also put up a good fight against any healthy eating plan you use as your weight-loss tactic—or any walking path, aerobics tape, weight-lifting class, or exercise program you use as your fat-burning weapon. Don't despair; your eating and exercise efforts will prevail as long as you hold the line and keep them coming. Eventually your fat cells will lose their competitive edge, but until then, they will fight with all their might to protect their precious gold mine of fat.

"But that doesn't make sense!" protested one of my clients, Sue Ellen. "I'm not pregnant anymore, so I don't need the help of my fat cells. Their job is done; they have nothing to protect any longer. So why won't my fat cells let me lose weight?" Because they still think you may need their truckload of stored fat from pregnancy. From a fat cell's perspective, it makes complete sense to hold on to their stored fat. Now that you've delivered your baby, they know that their job is only *half* done. As estrogen levels plummet, your fat cells are called upon to help produce some estrogen for you. It will take weeks for your ovaries to start secreting estrogen again, so your fat cells come to your aid by manufacturing some estrogen to help balance your hormones, lift your mood, strengthen your bones, improve your sleep, and lubricate your vagina. As I discuss in later chapters, estrogen levels can drop so low after delivery that you may feel like you've entered menopause instead of motherhood.

And as your estrogen levels are dropping, another hormone, prolactin, is rising. Prolactin is your milk-producing hormone for lactation, and it signals your fat cells to hold on tight to their stored fat. If you're breastfeeding, you need those stored calories to help produce milk. And that's why most studies have found that breastfeeding mothers weigh more than bottle-feeding mothers. No, this is not a typo. Even though weight loss has been used as a strong motivator to choose the breast over the bottle, little research exists to support the link between lactation and fat loss. And many of the studies that do show an unquestionable link were done years ago on rats. That's great if you want to be a thin rat, but the last I checked, most women had few, if any, similarities to rats (some men, on the other hand, may be direct descendants). The tried-and-true motivators for breastfeeding are nutrients and antibodies for your baby and oxytocin for you. Oxytocin is a hormone released from suckling that contracts the uterus and helps to shrink it back to its prepregnant size. It also makes its way up to the brain to help counteract stress and depression. That's why breastfeeding moms are less likely to experience the baby blues—and more likely to report an easier transition into motherhood.

So your postpartum fat cells are initially concerned about your estrogen levels and milk production, but they also have ongoing fears to address before they decide it's safe to release some fat and let you lose weight: What if you continue to breastfeed for many months? What if you get pregnant again soon? What if a famine hits in the near future? And their biggest fear: What if you get pregnant while you're still breastfeeding when that famine hits? "Oh no," they frantically conclude. "Better keep this fat under lock and key until we are absolutely sure that she doesn't need us any longer."

Even when your hormones are back to normal levels and you're no longer breastfeeding, your postpartum fat cells' survival mechanism is so advanced and strong that other factors join in to make sure they stay pleasantly plump:

- **Your metabolism is lower.** It may be 15–25 percent lower now than when you were pregnant. This means that your ability to burn calories is 15–25 percent lower. And if you can't burn them, you store them, which makes your fat cells very happy. Your metabolism will rise back to normal levels over the next six months, but until then, your fat cells are in control.

- **Your ability to burn fat while exercising is lower.** While you're sweating and panting at the gym, pool, or power-walking class, your fat cells are yawning with boredom and ready to take a nap. Even before you got pregnant, your fat cells tried to resist exercise; women generally take twenty to thirty minutes longer than men to burn fat while working out. But now that you're postpartum, it may take months before your fat cells start to release any fat and catch up to your prepregnant fat-burning level.

- **Your leptin levels are lower.** Derived from a Greek word meaning "thin," leptin is a recently discovered hormone that increases your fat-burning potential and decreases your appetite. When leptin levels are high, it's easy to shrink your fat cells and lose weight. When leptin levels are low, your fat cells won't budge, no matter how hard you try. Don't worry, your leptin levels will naturally rise again after a few months. And no, you can't buy leptin pills at the pharmacy or health-food store. Not yet, anyway.

- **Your thyroid hormones may be lower.** Some women experience postpartum hypothyroidism for a few months after delivery, and an underactive thyroid leads to overactive fat cells. The thyroid hormones boost your metabolism, and when their levels are lower, your metabolism and ability to lose weight is lower, too.

And arm yourself for this one: With all of these factors working in your fat cells' favor, they not only stay large after you have your baby, some of them keep growing. Research at Louisiana State University has found that the fat cells in your arms keep expanding for three months after delivery. Maybe our arms were fast asleep while the lower body was pulling an all-nighter pushing and contracting during labor, and then it took them awhile to figure out that we weren't pregnant any longer.

After reading this section, I'm sure you now get the picture. Your postpartum fat cells closely resemble your pregnant fat cells. The fat storing enzymes that were stimulated during pregnancy stay active. And the fat cells that grew during pregnancy maintain most of their growth.

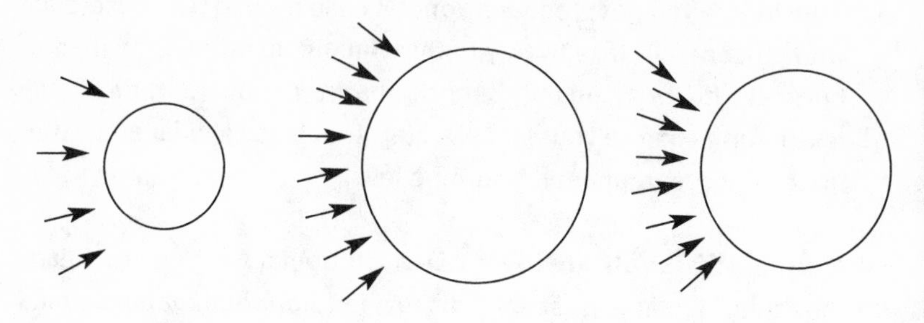

Before Pregnancy During Pregnancy After Pregnancy

"This explains everything!" exclaimed Maria. "Now I know why my clothes still don't fit, why my arms are jiggling, and why my abdomen still looks six months pregnant. But how long will my fat cells stay active? When will they turn off their survival mechanism? How long will it take for me to lose the weight?" Then she paused and looked at me with wide eyes. "I will lose the weight, won't I?"

I promise you that you will lose the weight. Your body doesn't want to carry all the excess weight from pregnancy. It's a strain on your heart, lungs, bones, and joints. And it's harmful to your health and longevity. Your body wants you to live long so that you can enjoy your children and future grandchildren in your later years. Rest assured that eventually your fat cells will have no choice but to cooperate with your efforts—as long as your efforts are nonthreatening and your timeline and expectations are realistic. It won't take six weeks or even six months to outsmart your postpartum fat cells. It took you nine months to gain the fat during pregnancy, and it will take most of you at least nine to twelve months to lose the fat afterward.

If you're six months postpartum, you're probably nodding your head in agreement, accepting the nine to twelve month fate of your fat cells because you've been living with their stubborn nature since the birth of your child. If you've just delivered your baby, you may be feeling discouraged before you even start trying to lose weight. I don't blame you; nine to twelve months seems like a lifetime away. But those months will fly by, and you have the advantage now of preparing yourself with patience, realistic expectations, and truthful facts. Honesty is always the best policy, even when it comes to the painfully slow and arduous weight loss in the postpartum months.

The Honest Facts About After-the-Baby Fat

Breastfeeding will melt away the fat in six weeks flat! Cut out the sugar and carbos after the baby and you'll be skinnier than ever before! Exercise will give you your body back! Get fit before you get pregnant and you'll remain fit throughout your pregnancy and into postpartum! Do crunches and your tummy will be flatter and firmer than ever! Take these fat-burning pills and you'll be back into your jeans in no time! Try this anticellulite lotion and your thighs will be as smooth as your baby's bottom! Follow this body-slimming program and you'll weigh less in six months than before you got pregnant!

These are just a few of the enthusiastic promises made in numerous postpartum books, articles, and promotional advertisements. Many women expect these promises to be fulfilled, only to then feel betrayed by their bodies when their jeans won't make it past their thighs, their stomachs won't flatten without the help of lycra-filled control-top pantyhose, and their cellulite won't disappear no matter what remedy they try.

Do you feel betrayed by your body? If you erroneously think that you should fit into your prepregnancy clothes within two months, you'll conclude that your body is a misfit. If you expect to weigh less after pregnancy than ever before in your adult life, you're expecting a miracle. And although miracles do sometimes happen, the probability of two occurring in one year is highly unlikely. Your body just performed an amazing miracle with the birth of your baby, and another one right now is simply out of the question.

If you can't believe the promises, and you can't expect a miracle—what can you expect your body to do in the months and years after your baby? I think it's time to set the record straight about postpartum weight. So here's the postpartum truth, the whole truth, and nothing but the truth.

- **Right after you delivered your baby, the scale dropped twelve incredible pounds** (seven plus pounds from the weight of your baby, three from the amniotic fluid, and two from your placenta). This may be the most weight you ever lost in one day, but you probably felt like you left the delivery room in the same condition you arrived. Your uterus was still expanded to its nine-month size, and you were still carrying twelve to twenty pounds of pregnancy fat.

- **In the first week or two, your newborn may lose more weight than you do.** Most babies lose 5–10 percent of their body weight in the first weeks following birth. Most new mothers lose 1–2 percent if they're lucky.

- **For the next six weeks, most of the weight you lose is extra fluid stored in your bloodstream and cells.** Those night sweats and frequent trips to the bathroom happen for a reason—to flush out the five pounds of fluid left over from pregnancy.

- **For the next month or so, most women only lose half a pound of fat per week.** The good news is that the bloatedness is gone and your uterus is back in place, but your fat cells are still there protecting you and refusing to shrink back to their prepregnancy state.

- **At the three- to six-month mark, your body finally starts speeding up the weight-loss process.** This is when your fat cells deem it safe to give up some of their extra fat. No famine has hit, you're not pregnant again, and if you're like most women, you've probably stopped breastfeeding. Less than 10 percent of us are still breastfeeding at six months. But don't think you'll drop all your weight in the sixth month; most women need another six months after that before their bodies resemble their prepregnant selves.

- **Breastfeeding is best for your baby, but not necessarily for your after-the-baby fat.** Most studies have found that women who breastfeed weigh more at six months than women who bottle-feed, but the length of time spent breastfeeding appears to be the real determining factor. The University of California at Davis found that six to twelve months is the weight loss ticket with breastfeeding. After six months, the fat stores are mobilized, and by a year breastfeeding moms weigh significantly less than bottle-feeding moms. But most new mothers stop breastfeeding well before a year. Of the 52 percent who choose to breastfeed, only 5 percent are doing it on their child's first birthday. So maybe breast-feeding does encourage weight loss, but we just aren't doing it long enough to reap the benefit.

- **Exercise may not melt away the fat on a brand-new mother.** I am such a strong advocate of exercise that it's very disconcerting for me not to be able to tell you that it's a weight-loss guarantee from the very beginning. Most studies have found that exercising in the first three months does not speed up weight loss. Women who walk daily weigh the same as those who stay at home and watch *Days of our Lives* daily. Remember, your fat cells want to hold on to their stored fat for estrogen production, breastfeeding, and a future pregnancy or famine. However, exercise is *not* a waste of time. You'll be preparing your fat cells to more efficiently release fat once they are ready—and they will be soon.

- **A million crunches may not tone your tummy in a timely fashion.** Your abdominal muscles have stretched by 300 percent, and time as well as effort is necessary for them to return to their original form. For most women, it takes about a year to get their tummies back in tip-top shape. If you had a C-section, those stomach muscles were cut as well as stretched and may never heal back to their tight, compact, prepregnancy, presurgery state. And in case you haven't heard, sit-ups don't shrink fat cells. They tone the muscles underneath the fat, but the burning sensation you feel while doing them doesn't mean they are burning away the fat. Only aerobic exercise burns fat: walking, running, swimming, cycling, dancing, stair stepping, or any other activity that uses your buttocks and thighs in a rhythmical, nonstop movement.

- **You may have to accept a few extra pounds of fat.** The average woman holds on to two to five pregnancy pounds for years after delivery. Why? Nobody knows for sure, but your fat cells may be banking away some calories for you when your baby hits the toddler years. When your mobile, energetic little one doesn't sit still, neither do you. One interesting study had professional athletes follow toddlers around for a day, mimicking their behavior. Not only did they burn hundreds of extra calories, they found it more exhausting than their training schedules. They tired within two hours of tailing a toddler.

- **Even if you do lose every ounce of weight you gained, your body shape may be different.** Your hips may be permanently wider, your waist less defined than it used to be, and your thighs slightly larger than before. Many women have said to me, "I've lost all the weight, but I still can't fit into some of my clothes!" And I reply, "Then it's time to buy some new clothes to complement your new body." And your new body can be fitter, sexier, and stronger than ever before.

- **A lean and fit body before pregnancy does not guarantee a lean and fit body after.** Research has found that fitness level, body fat, and weight before getting pregnant are *not* determining factors for weight loss after delivery. This is great news for some of you who haven't moved a muscle for the last decade. For those of you who have always been fitness divas, it means you may have to put in just as much time and effort as couch potatoes.

- **Dieting during the postpartum months will only cause your fat cells to hold on to more of their fat for a longer period of time.** Women who diet retain twice as much weight as women who don't—and are still holding on to their pregnancy weight well after a year.

"But how else am I going to lose the weight?" asked Julie after I shared these honest facts. "I'm just about to start a high protein diet because the diet pills I tried didn't work. I can't wait for my fat cells to decide when it's safe for me to lose weight. I can't wait months for exercise to work. I can't wait a year for my body to lose all the weight. I have to lose it now!" Like Julie, you may not be in agreement with your fat cells' timeline for weight loss, but dieting won't speed it up; it will only delay weight loss. *If you diet today, you'll have to deal with even more stubborn postpartum fat cells tomorrow.*

Diet Traps That Keep You Fat

In a society that worships thinness and condones dieting, I realize that it's difficult to accept the fact that diet books, programs, drinks, and pills won't work. So let's spend some time convincing you beyond any reasonable doubt that dieting isn't the solution to postpartum weight loss. It didn't work before you got pregnant, and it's definitely not going to work now. I've had clients spend hours arguing with me, "Yes, dieting did work for me. Before I got pregnant, I went on over a dozen diets, and they worked every single time." If dieting really worked, you'd only have to go on one and be forever thin. You may have lost weight for a few weeks or months by dieting, but then you gained it back and had to go on another diet. If you go on another diet now in your postpartum months, you may not even have the fleeting, short-term satisfaction of temporary weight loss. Here's why:

- **Your metabolism is already reduced by 15–25 percent—and dieting can make it drop even lower.** Following a one-thousand-calorie diet has been found to cut metabolism by as much as 40 percent. So if you thought your metabolism was sluggish before, restrictive dieting can make it resemble that of a sloth.

- **Your fat cells are already waiting for a potential famine—and dieting tells them that their wait is over.** Your body doesn't know the difference between a real famine and a self-imposed dieting famine, so when you cut the calories, your fat cells go into survival mode to protect their stored fat.

- **You've already lost some muscle during labor and delivery—and dieting can make you lose even more.** While your body is protecting its stored fat, it's sacrificing muscle for needed energy. The University of California at Davis had new mothers diet for eight weeks, and found that they lost one-and-a-half pounds of muscle as a result. Losing one-and-a-half pounds of muscle may not sound like a lot, but it will reduce your metabolism by seventy-five calories a day and increase your weight by up to eight pounds in one year.

- **Your leptin levels are already low—and dieting can cause them to drop even lower.** The more you reduce calories, the more you'll reduce leptin. The result: your appetite soars and your fat-burning potential wanes. No wonder we gain all the weight back with dieting; a slower metabolism and lower leptin levels guarantee it.

- **You're already less than happy with your postbaby shape—and dieting can make you detest it.** An Australian study found that those new mothers who dieted had greater body dissatisfaction than those women who didn't. And the more dissatisfied you are with your body, the more likely you are to sabotage your efforts at weight loss. Those women who disliked their bodies were least likely to exercise and eat healthfully and most likely to develop an eating disorder.

You may think that eating disorders only affect vulnerable young teenagers or adult women with traumatic histories such as physical or sexual abuse, but the University of Oxford in England found that pregnancy was one of the strongest life events to trigger an eating disorder. And combined with weight preoccupation and dieting obsessions, the eating disorder dominoes can be set in motion. While pregnant, gaining weight was probably acceptable because it was for the baby. Our beautifully growing belly distracted us from our hips, thighs, and buttocks. But once our babies were born, our weights became our nemeses and our bodies became our opponents in the diet war.

Think about your own current situation: You're frustrated with your weight, your clothes don't fit, the mirror is not your friend, and the bathroom scale is an outright enemy. Innocently enough, you start a diet, then your frustration makes you take it up a notch by skipping meals, cutting out all fat, eliminating whole food groups, taking weight loss pills, fearing calories—and then possibly purging calories through starvation, exercise, laxatives, or even vomiting. I've witnessed this sequence of events in thousands of women. A simple diet becomes an obsession, which eventually can turn into an eating disorder.

I must take a moment to get serious and personal. Eating disorders destroy lives—yours and those around you. If you're starving yourself with anorexia or binging and purging with bulimia, I urge you to seek immediate treatment. Your eating disorder may have begun recently as a result of pregnancy, or it may have begun years ago and continued throughout your pregnancy. Despite fertility problems, some women with eating disorders do get pregnant, and most manage to keep their vomiting or starvation a secret. Although it's impossible to hide a severe case of anorexia, many borderline anorexics successfully conceal their disorder by saying that they "are thin because they have a fast metabolism" or that they "eat very low fat for their health" or that they "aren't eating because they just ate." And even though there is a greater chance of premature birth, low birth weight, and stillbirths, many anorexic women deliver healthy, vital babies. It's amazing what a woman's body will do to ensure the health of her baby—even when calories and nutrients are lacking.

With the binge–purge disorder, bulimia, it's much easier to keep the vomiting a secret in the privacy of the bathroom with air freshener and toilet cleaner handy. Bulimics are usually normal weight or even slightly overweight, so no one would suspect their unhealthy behavior. And during early pregnancy, many bulimics have shared with me that morning sickness was a convenient cover for their continued vomiting. But as pregnancy progresses, studies have found that 75 percent of bulimics successfully stop their binge–purge behavior for the health of their developing babies. Unfortunately, most start up again once the baby is born, and half of the women vomit more postpartum than they did prepregnancy.

But the damaging effects of eating disorders do not stop once the baby is born. The rituals of binging and purging take an immense amount of time and energy away from caring for your baby, and a starvation diet decreases the quantity and quality of breast milk. Eating-disordered mothers have also been found to project their own weight preoccupations and food fears onto their children. In extreme cases, restrictive infant feeding leads to failure to thrive where babies are lethargic, unresponsive, and developmentally delayed because of a lack of calories and fat. In most other cases, mothers with eating problems are more likely to bring up children with eating problems—children who fear food and are underweight, or children who eat compulsively and are overweight.

Only you can judge whether or not the preceding discussion of eating disorders applies to you. You may think that you'd never throw up because you hate the thought, or that you'd never starve yourself because you love food too much—but you may still dislike your body, restrict your eating, diet the first Monday of every month, forbid your favorite foods, and feel guilty when you do indulge and eat a real meal. You may not have an eating disorder, but you may be a *disordered eater,* meaning that you have an unhealthy relationship with food and your body. Before you protest, please be advised that I am not singling you out. Most women in this country are disordered eaters: 90 percent of us diet, 96 percent dislike our bodies, 80 percent fear weight gain, and 60 percent feel guilty after eating our favorite foods. We've grown up with an unrealistically thin ideal and the culture of dieting. We've matured into adults thinking that dieting, body dissatisfaction, and food fears are a normal part of being a woman. Well, there is nothing normal about waking up every morning hating your body, eating salad with fat-free dressing every day for lunch, or avoiding any event that calls for a bathing suit. *There is nothing normal about denying your body nourishment and denying yourself eating pleasure.*

My work with women is to help them free themselves from dieting and disordered eating. Oftentimes, this means convincing them that they are dieting, even though they say they aren't. With the antidieting/body acceptance movement now in full swing, women are encouraged and expected to speak out against the thin ideal and join together to put an end to dieting. To diet is to turn your back on fellow females and this worthy and necessary antidieting mission. So, most of us don't "diet" any longer, instead we "watch what we eat" or "eat lightly" or "eat low fat" or "eat mostly fruits and vegetables for our health." All socially acceptable ways of healthy eating, but on further reflection, all socially acceptable ways of destructive dieting. We may not be consuming foul smelling cabbage soup, peeling dozens of grapefruits, sipping pasty liquid meals, or popping fat-burning diet pills, but many of us are still dieting, just the same. If your primary reason for watching what you eat, eating lightly, eating low fat, or eating healthy, is quick weight loss—*then you're dieting*. It's just disguised under the sheep's clothing of healthy eating behaviors.

In the past, specially designed diets for postpartum women included some outrageous premises. There was the Baby Food Diet, where you eat what your baby eats to lose weight; the Pacifier Diet, where you suck on sugar-free lollipops all day long; and the Celery and Celibacy Diet, where avoiding another pregnancy and avoiding every food but celery were the goals. I'm sure some women temporarily lost weight on these diets, but they also lost a lot of enjoyment from eating and life. All celery and no sex makes Jill a dull girl, so to speak.

Today, I think we know better than to try some laughable diet gimmick to shed those unwanted postpartum pounds, but we could still use some smarts when it comes to outsmarting our postpartum fat cells. No diet by any name, crazy or credible, is going to help you slim down and lose weight. The only way to permanently lose weight is to do the opposite of dieting—*eating*. In the next chapter, I'll share with you all the strategies to successfully outsmart postpartum fat, but the most important one is knowledge and an appreciation of your postbaby fat cells. Yes, at first glance, they are strong and stubborn, pesky and persnickety. But on a deeper level they are savvy and smart and perfectly predictable. *They are protecting themselves in order to protect you.*

THOSE PERFECTLY PREDICTABLE POSTPARTUM POUNDS

You now have a full understanding of your postpartum fat cells. To know them may not be to love them, but at least you can respect them for the benefits they are giving you. *They are not out to get you; they are out to save you.* Your fat cells are doing exactly what they should be doing: holding on to their fat in case of an unexpected famine or unplanned pregnancy, or both, in which case they act like kamikaze pilots who will fight to the death to protect their stored fat, and therefore, you. And the particular areas of your body that are holding on to the most fat are doing it for important reasons:

- **Your hips**—because they contain the most concentrated number of fat cells, and therefore, provide the greatest reserve of calories for an emergency and the best mode of transportation for your baby. The bigger your hips, the easier it is to carry your infant around.

- **Your stomach**—because the fat cells around your waist have the ability to produce some estrogen for you as well as the ability to provide a comfy pillow for your little one to nap on.

- **Your breasts**—because they are made primarily of fat and need that fat to produce milk. What lover would cry all the way home because he couldn't wait to get hold of one of your breasts? Need I say more about how important your breasts are to your baby?

If you're still having a difficult time appreciating your plump postpartum fat cells, consider this: You'd be struggling to lose much more weight if your fat cells didn't enthusiastically volunteer to grow during pregnancy. Let me explain. If you stored the needed calories during pregnancy as carbohydrates instead of fat, you would have gained more than twice the weight and would be struggling to lose twenty-five to forty-five pounds instead of twelve to twenty right now. *Your fat cells were actually doing you a favor when they came to the rescue during pregnancy.* Storing calories as fat was the most efficient way of gaining weight without putting too much strain on your body or the bathroom scale. It also provided the best protection and greatest health benefit for you and your baby. Without it, your child could never have been born.

Let me ask you a question: If you were to go back in time, would you not have gotten pregnant if you knew the effect it would have on your fat cells and body shape? Most women I have posed this question to immediately answered, "No way! Having a baby was the most important thing I've done in my life. My baby is much more important than my body." Others have had to contemplate the question for just a few seconds and after a long pause, answered, "I wouldn't trade my baby for a thin body in a million years, but I would like both, a beautiful baby *and* a beautiful body."

You *can* have both—a new, beautiful baby and a new, beautiful body. You don't have to stop taking care yourself when you start taking care of your baby. You don't have to give up looking good to be a good mother. And you certainly don't have to appear matronly to be maternal. All it takes is a little patience, a lot of support, and a few effective strategies to encourage your postpartum fat cells to shrink back to their prepregnancy size. And this book will give you all the encouragement, support, and knowledge you need to outsmart your fat cells once and for all.

Chapter Two

If You Can't Beat Them, Join Them

Imagine yourself for a moment on a battlefield waving a white flag at your fat cells, calling a truce, inviting them to sit down to some peace talks, and then shaking hands with your newly formed ally. Picture working together toward a common goal of making you fit and healthy, jointly brainstorming to come up with the most effective strategies to keep both parties satisfied, and then implementing those strategies with unanimous support and commitment. What would happen? You'd find that this peacekeeping approach works a whole lot better than fighting a useless battle where you're outnumbered thirty billion to one.

As women, we're much more likely to try to come to a peaceful solution in any potential war situation, at home or abroad. We prefer compromise over conflict, communication over cannons, and words over weapons. Why fight, we think, when you can sit down and come up with a reasonable compromise that makes everyone happy?

So, why not do what women do best? Try to avoid a long, drawn-out war by making peace with your fat cells. Sit down and have a heart-to-heart talk with them, analyze the situation from every possible angle, figure out an amicable solution, and put forth a reasonable resolution. I guarantee you, it's not only possible; it's been done. Thousands of my clients have made peace with their fat cells, relying on them as a much-needed ally in the battle of postbaby bulge.

"Not my fat cells!" argued Margaret. "They have been enemy number one for the past twenty years. We can't work together as allies; we've been dueling for decades like the Hatfields and McCoys. There's no way we can communicate, never mind live amicably in the same body." If, like Margaret, you've been fighting your fat cells since puberty, let me remind you that after decades of fighting, the actual Hatfields and McCoys are now on speaking terms, and some are even friends. After all these years, they have found out that they have a lot more in common than fighting and feuding.

Where it really counts, you'll find that you and your fat cells have much in common, too. For example, your fat cells really don't want you to diet, and you'd rather not starve yourself with unsatisfying foods either. Your fat cells don't want you to overexercise, and you'd rather not spend hours at the gym sweating and panting (even if you had the time). Your fat cells want you to lose the weight, and you desperately want to lose the weight. Your major area of disagreement is in the timing of that weight loss. Your fat cells want to lose weight slowly; a year sounds reasonable to them. You, on the other hand, want to lose weight quickly; next week would be good, tomorrow would be great. If you want to keep peace and lose the weight, you have no choice but to accept your fat cells' weight loss schedule. They have the upper hand in determining your weight loss, and that hand is holding the timer. If you try to lose all your pregnancy weight in three or four months, they'll call off the peace treaty and retaliate. If you diet or overexercise, they'll think you're violating the demilitarized zone and will counterattack. If you attempt to speed up the weight-loss process, they will slow it down even more—and years from now when your child enters kindergarten, you'll still be carrying around those last ten pounds as a constant reminder that you opted for war over peace.

Think about what's really important to you: losing the weight quickly or losing the weight, period. If you can you accept losing weight slowly over a year without starvation or overexercising—and keeping it off forever—then you can make peace with your fat cells. Just about every woman I've come across says that she can accept it, even if she mumbles the words through gritted teeth. We all know that in the long run, it really doesn't matter if we lose the weight in three months, six months, or twelve months. *What matters is that we lose the weight.*

My goal is to help you and your fat cells successfully lose the weight by finding the middle ground where you both get what you want—where your fat cells get to protect you without being threatened, and you get to lose the weight without gaining it back. To achieve this goal, you need a peaceful plan of action to work with your fat cells, one that puts an end to the fighting from this day forth.

YOUR POSTPARTUM PEACE PLAN

"So, you want me to do the sixties thing and 'make love, not war'?" asked Sarah when I first explained the Postpartum Peace Plan. Well, kind of. You may not necessarily fall in love with your fat cells, and sex may be the last thing on your mind, but you can have a mutually satisfying relationship where each knows how to please the other. Your fat cells know that the ultimate pleasure they could give you is to shrink back down to their prepregnancy size. You know that the ultimate pleasure you could give your fat cells is to let them do their own thing on their own schedule and not force them to shrink with dieting. So in the spirit of the sixties, I asked Sarah to join the anti-dieting movement and burn her diet books like her mother burned her bras in the women's movement. And she quickly replied, "No thanks. I'm a yuppie, not a hippie like my mom was. I may quietly put my diet books in storage, but I won't actively torch them in protest on my front lawn."

Obviously, the sixties analogy didn't work for Sarah, but she did eventually come to a compromise with her fat cells by agreeing not to diet, and by acquiring the patience to lose weight slowly. And then one day, she walked into my office with a tie-dyed shirt and faded blue jeans announcing, "Your Postpartum Peace Plan worked. These were my favorite jeans before I got pregnant, and I'm wearing them today because I made love, not war, and gave peace a chance."

Are you ready to give the Postpartum Peace Plan a chance? Before reading this book, your postpartum weight loss plan probably focused on dieting. In fact, two out of every three women say that they planned to step off the delivery table dieting. Did you? Are you? If you're either currently dieting or plan to start soon, you definitely need this plan. And that's just about every woman since 50 percent are dieting right this very moment and another 30 percent plan to start on Monday.

So, first things first. Before you even hear about the plan, I want you to let your fat cells know that you will not violate the peace treaty by going on any kind of diet today, tomorrow, next week, or next month. And the best way of informing them is to actively remove dieting and all its paraphernalia from your life. So, get up right now and:

- Go into your bathroom, pick up that scale, and put it in the trash, garage, or closet. As long as you're getting on the scale, you'll be functioning in the dieting mode. The scale will only remind you of how slowly you're losing weight, and you'll be tempted to diet to speed up the weight loss process. You can't speed it up; your fat cells are in the driver's seat. And just like the saying "a watched pot never boils," a watched scale never budges. Who can get excited about a quarter pound loss here or a half-pound loss there? You'll be surprised to find that you lose weight more quickly when you have no idea how much weight you're losing.

- Go to your bookcase, pack up all your diet books, and put them in the recycling bin—the old and the new, the ones you tried ten years ago, and the ones you haven't even opened yet. And don't forget the one in your beach bag that your mother gave you last summer before she knew you were pregnant—and the one in your car trunk that your mother-in-law gave you when she found out you were pregnant.

- Go into your kitchen and toss out the overpriced prepackaged "diet" foods left over from your last weight loss attempt, the diet soft drinks, the liquid meal replacers, and any food in the cupboard or refrigerator that you eat only when you're on a diet. It may be diet Jell-O, cottage cheese, or rice cakes, but whatever it is, replace it with a tasty, satisfying, nondiet food.

- Go into your medicine cabinet and dump the diet pills, fat-burning supplements, and weight loss herbs—including the phen-fen you may have taken before it was taken off the market, the chromium picolinate you may have taken before you got pregnant, and the amphetamines you may have taken when you were much younger and didn't know any better.

- Go into your closet and get rid of those ten-year-old pants, dresses, and suits that are two sizes too small, but you've been saving for that nonexistent day of dieting success. If you couldn't fit into them before you got pregnant, you certainly won't be able to now.

How did it feel to actively remove dieting and its baggage from your life? Stephanie thought it was one of the most freeing experiences of her life. But after she "cleansed her house" and made it a "diet-free dwelling," she had a pressing question, "Now what? If dieting isn't a part of my postpartum weight loss plan, what is?"

Your Postpartum Peace Plan has nothing to do with counting calories, limiting fat, banning bread, or eliminating sugar. It has nothing to do with eating for your body type, your blood type, or your personality type. It was not designed by a famous actress, personal trainer to the stars, or Oprah's chef. It was put together by a forty-year-old, postpartum woman with a graduate degree in nutrition who knows exactly what you're going through. I am in the same place as you are right now. I know your frustrations, struggles, needs, hopes, and wants. And I know what works and what doesn't. Restriction, deprivation, and starvation don't work. Slowly integrating eating and exercise strategies designed specifically for your postpartum body does. Professionally, I know the Postpartum Peace Plan works because I've used it with thousands of clients. Personally, I know it works because I'm following it myself.

So what exactly is this Postpartum Peace Plan? First, and most important, it is a timeline for change, outlining what to focus on from the first six weeks through the next six years. The needs of a mother who just had her baby last week are very different from one who had her child six months or a year ago. The willingness (or lack thereof) of your fat cells to shrink in the first month is very different from their willingness in the sixth month. The lifestyle of a brand-spanking-new mother is very different from that of a six-year veteran.

- **The first six weeks.** Your fat cells are resting after a job well done, and you should be, too. Other than the natural weight loss that occurs after delivery, there's really nothing you can do to make your fat cells release fat anyway. So relax and take it easy. Don't worry about anything except healing your body and bonding with your baby. It's a magical time you don't want to miss. It's also a major recovery time, especially if you had a C-section. Your overall focus should be on getting the rest you need and eating as well as you did during your pregnancy. A healthy diet will not only give your body the strength to heal, it will also give your breasts a sufficient milk supply to nourish your little one. Once you've achieved a healthy diet, sleeping is your next priority during these early weeks. The oft-given advice to "sleep when your baby sleeps" should be heeded, because your baby won't sleep when you do.

- **The next six weeks.** Your fat cells are slowly waking up from their after-birth rest, and you're waking up to the after-birth reality of your body and your life. All of a sudden, you feel the pressure of taking care of your baby and tackling your weight. Your mother has gone home, your partner is back to his hectic work schedule, your friends are no longer stopping by with casseroles and gifts, and your doctor says you're fully recovered and can start exercising and having sex again. Eeeek! You're probably not feeling up to either, but would more likely choose the par course over intercourse—if you had the energy or the time. Most of your life is still consumed (and will be for the next eighteen years) with caring for your newborn, taking care of your other kids, cooking meals, doing the laundry—and juggling dozens of other responsibilities, including work, even though you're still technically on maternity leave. How can you have an eating schedule when you have no schedule? How can you find the time to exercise when you have no time? How can you make losing weight a priority when other priorities are more important? These are what I call the "beg, borrow, and steal" weeks. Beg for any help you can get, borrow babysitting time, and steal any minute you can for you.

- **The next six months.** Your fat cells are wide-awake and fully functioning. They are willing to release fat, albeit slowly, as long as they don't feel threatened. And you will slowly establish an eating and exercise routine that works with the realities of your lifestyle. Some of you will be going back to work full-time, others part-time. Some of you will be at home caring for your infant; others will be at home caring for your twin infants, toddler, and preschooler. Some of you will be juggling car pools, soccer games, birthday parties, PTA meetings, and board meetings; others will be juggling an exhausting number of unending responsibilities as a single mother. Whatever your life situation, this six-month block is your window of opportunity to outsmart your postpartum fat cells. And while you're peacefully encouraging them to shrink, you may have to outsmart some other postpartum annoyances such as hair loss, stretch marks, varicose veins, urinary incontinence, and debilitating fatigue.

- **The next six years and beyond.** Your fat cells will stay outsmarted unless you get pregnant again, become a wet nurse, or enter perimenopause. Since becoming a wet nurse is probably out of the question, another baby or the next stage of female passage is more probable, and I'll help you prepare for these weight-changing events. As your children are growing older, this is also the time to set a pro-eating, body-accepting example for them to follow. With young girls entering the world of dieting and body dissatisfaction as early as age eight, it's vital to create a safe haven in your home by becoming a nondieting role model and thereby balancing the outside media messages urging your children to pursue thinness.

For yourself and your children, it's best to start your Postpartum Peace Plan during the first six weeks, but it doesn't matter where you are in the postpartum timeline. *It's never too late to outsmart your postpartum fat cells.* If you didn't shrink them in the first year, you can deflate them in the fifth. If you've been in a never-ending war with your fat cells since your child was born, you can end that battle today and maintain peaceful relations from this day forth. How? With the five principles for postpartum peace.

Pamper yourself
Eat with a regular meal schedule
Actively move your body
Calm your stress
Embrace your new body

1. **Pamper yourself.** In other countries, women are cared for by family and friends for two to three months after delivery. In this country, we're lucky if we get two days in the hospital (at least you can rest), then it's home to the dirty dishes, loads of laundry, and twenty-four-hour infant care. Since it's too late to relocate to Asia or Africa, you have to redesign your life to include some pampering for you. I'm not asking you to care for your children less; I'm encouraging you to care for yourself more. Pampering yourself can take many different forms: resting when you're tired, hiring a sitter when you need a break, inviting a friend over when you need to socialize, eating a snack when you're hungry, getting a massage when you feel tense, or laughing when your spirit needs a lift. It's been documented that mothers respond to their infants' needs at least once a minute. If we could respond to our own needs at least once a day, we'd be making headway. And when you do something that makes *you* feel good, you'll feel more balanced and have more energy to care for your baby and yourself.

2. **Eat with a regular meal schedule.** Fueling your body on a consistent, regular basis is vital for all your concerns: healing your body, fighting fatigue, producing breast milk, alleviating sadness, balancing moods, growing your hair back, and of course, losing weight. But what should you eat to outsmart your postpartum fat cells? The answer is not cutting out the fat. And it's not cutting out the carbs. It's eating everything—fat, carbohydrates, and protein—and research has proven it. Those people who lose the weight and keep it off do not cut out food groups; they eat *all* foods. What they do cut out is large portions. *If your meals are*

small, you will become a smaller postpartum woman. The Stockholm Pregnancy and Weight Development Study evaluated one thousand four hundred women and found that those who lost the most postpartum weight had a regular meal schedule with a small breakfast, a midmorning snack, a small lunch, a midafternoon snack, and a small dinner. *Meal size and meal schedule separated the losers from the gainers.*

3. **Actively move your body.** Exercise may not be the weight loss answer in the first couple of months, but it is the solution for the rest of your life. The University of Michigan found that postpartum women who made exercise a part of their lives lost 25 percent more weight than those who exercised sporadically or not at all. Three times a week is all it takes to boost your metabolism, build strength, and burn fat. And to tighten those loose abdominal muscles and tone your other muscles, crunches and weight lifting are vital. But the benefits of exercise go beyond muscle repair and fat loss. More postpartum women say that they exercise more for stress reduction than for weight reduction.

4. **Calm your stress.** Stress is the most frequently used word in a mother's vocabulary, and it's the culprit that prohibits us from achieving optimal life happiness and optimal body weight. When we're stressed out (when aren't we?), we stress out our fat cells and they respond by shutting down fat release and turning on storage again. That's why stress and postpregnancy are not a compatible mix and that's why we have to learn how to calm our stress response. The National Weight Control Registry, the largest organization tracking weight loss success, has discovered that those with effective stress management skills are more likely to lose the weight and keep it off. In chapter 5, I'll share with you ten stress busters to help you bust through the barriers of postpartum weight loss, many of which are out of the ordinary. For example, I encourage the overuse of paper products: paper plates,

paper cups, and paper towels (if it makes you feel better, you can always recycle). Fewer dishes to wash and less laundry to do means more time for you—to exercise, read, nap, or relax. And I discourage writing too many thank-you notes (my mother would be very disappointed). It takes a lot less time to say "thank you" than to sit down and write it on paper. The most appreciated words spoken to me during the first few months were, "You don't have to send me a thank-you note, just thank me now." I vow to grant those same calming words to others.

5. **Embrace your new body.** Every step of the way, you have to accept and respect your body to lose weight. If you don't, you won't take the time to treat it well with food, fitness, and self-care. At the beginning, you may easily embrace your body for its miraculous life-giving ability. The fact that I made it through labor and lived to tell about it was enough for me to revel for weeks in my body's strength and power. But as the weeks and months pass, you're bound to get frustrated with your body for not losing the weight and regaining its shape. And if it never regains its shape, you may never be able to find joy in your body again. I don't want that to happen. *This is your body, the only one you'll ever have.* It delivered a beautiful baby for you, it keeps your baby fed, warm, and safe, it moves you to where you need to go each day, and it sees, smells, and feels the world around you. Even if you do lose all the weight, it will still be a new, different body to embrace. After what it went through with pregnancy and birth, it could never be the same old, boring body. It now has wisdom, strength, and experience that the old body could only dream of.

This is how these five principles will help you make peace with your body, your fat cells, and your new roller-coaster life as a mother. When you present these PEACE principles to your fat cells, they will be nodding their heads in agreement, eager to sign off on the plan because:

- When you pamper your body by taking care of it, they have less to worry about.
- When you eat with a regular meal schedule, they forget about a possible famine.
- When you actively move your body, they allow some fat to move out.
- When you calm your stress, they have less to get stressed out about.
- When you embrace your body, they feel welcomed instead of threatened and will help you reach a new, comfortable, healthy weight that's right for you.

Embracing your body may be the most difficult principle to put into practice. Clients have asked with tears in their eyes, "How can I embrace my body when I can't even bear to look at it in the mirror? How can I feel good about my body when I feel fat all the time? How can I accept my body when I still have twenty pounds to lose? How can I respect my body when it won't let me fit into my size eight wardrobe?" You *can* and *will* when you have a clear, realistic picture of what to expect when you're no longer expecting.

Great Weight Expectations

How much weight do you expect to lose? What do you expect your body to look like? And most important: Do you think your expectations are realistic?

If you're like most postpartum women, your initial answer is that you expect to lose all the weight and look exactly like you did before you got pregnant. And even as you speak those words, you probably know up front that your expectations are unreasonable. In fact, 72 percent of us fear that we won't reach our weight goals before we even start trying to achieve them. That fear is our subconscious telling us to jump ship now and reassess our weight goals before it's

Expectation	Real Life Experience
I expected to be a little out of shape for a few weeks, but nothing that a little exercise couldn't take care of.	I was a walking bowl of Jell-O for months and even a lot of exercise couldn't stop the jiggle. I went from mother-to-be to mother-to-be-fat, and I'm still there.
I thought I'd use maternity leave to exercise twice as much as I ever have before, and I'd be back to normal by the time I went back to work at three months.	Maternity leave was a misnomer. I barely left the house and spent most of my time breastfeeding in my rocker. When I went back to work, nothing was back to normal, not my life or my body. I had to buy a whole new business wardrobe two sizes larger, and finally had to redefine my definition of normal.
I wanted to weigh what I did when I was eighteen years old, proving that pregnancy wouldn't get the best of my body.	I was thirty-eight, not eighteen, and couldn't turn back the clock twenty years no matter what I did. Pregnancy did get the best of my body, but it was the best thing I ever did.
Weight was never a problem for me, so I thought, no problem, the fat will melt away on its own.	Was I in for the shock of my life! Not only did the fat not melt away, it congealed as cellulite all over my body.
I expected to show all my girlfriends that I could get back to my old, fit self quicker than they did.	I didn't show my face or body in public for months until I realized that postpartum weight loss was not a competition, and that I was losing weight at the same pace as they did.
I really thought I could make myself look just like Cindy Crawford after she had a baby—model-thin within weeks.	I didn't look like Cindy Crawford before I got pregnant, so how could I look like her after? But I studied her photos with envy every day.

too late. But we don't listen and try anyway, thinking we can beat the odds and defy Mother Nature. Before you try, fail, and find yourself frustrated with your body and yourself, learn from other women who have gone before you. What they expected was not even close to what they experienced—and their unrealistic expectations gave them the postpartum body blues.

Let's take a moment to discuss celebrity pregnancies—it seems like every actress and model is having or recently had a baby. I'm happy for them, but their experiences can make us miserable. They seem to look like a million bucks at nine months pregnant, and then look like they never had a child on their first public appearance after delivery. The public display of pregnancy all started with Demi Moore in the buff on the cover of *Vanity Fair,* and then quite buffed as G. I. Jane shortly thereafter. Since then, we've watched Elle MacPherson, Annette Bening, Melanie Griffith, Heather Locklear, Catherine Zeta-Jones, Christie Brinkley, Madonna, Pamela Anderson, Cindy Crawford, and dozens more showing off their big tummies one day and their flat tummies the next.

Speaking of Cindy, a recent *People* magazine poll points to her as the woman we most aspire to look like. Who wouldn't want to look like her? But what real life mother could? Granted, she told *USA Weekend* that she has to live with "a little swimsuit jiggle," but most of us common folk have to live with so much jiggle that we might never be seen in a swimsuit in public again. When she's out in public, you can bet that she doesn't leave the house without a professional hair and makeup job, while we rush out without a stitch of makeup, often without even combing our hair. She may have bags under her eyes large enough to carry her child, too, but we'd never know it with the miracle concealer amply applied. She may be losing her hair, too, but we'd never know it with her volumizer shampooed, moussed hair blow-dried to perfection. Maybe we'd have these appearance-enhancing beauty products, too, if we had the money and a personal shopper at our beck and call twenty-four hours a day.

The who's who of celebrity mamas are surrounded by an entourage of worker bees. They have personal trainers to whip them back into shape, professional chefs to whip up delicious, nutritious low-fat meals, and full-time nannies to whisk away the kids while they get facials, body wraps, pedicures, and massages, and perhaps while they sneak away to the plastic surgeon for a little nip, tuck, and suck here and there to get rid of the loose skin, stretch marks, and extra fat. Whether or not your goal is to look like a model who had a model pregnancy and a model recovery, just seeing these model mamas is enough to send us into a spiral of body dissatisfaction. *What we see in magazines is worlds apart from what we see when we look in the mirror. And what we expect from our bodies is far from what we actually experience.*

The greater the difference between what you expect and what you experience, the lower your self-esteem and body image. One study found that postpartum women whose actual weights were higher than what they expected had the greatest body dissatisfaction and the lowest self-esteem. And most women were at least ten pounds away from their expected goals—except those women who were over thirty-five. Older women, not younger women as you might suspect, were more likely to reach their weight goals. Not because they lost more weight in the postpartum months, but because they had more realistic goals to begin with.

So, let me ask you again: How much weight do you expect to lose? What do you expect your body to look like? And are your expectations realistic? The best advice I can give you is to erase any and all expectations from your mind, and instead wait and see what happens to your weight. If you choose to turn the other cheek to this advice and hold on tight to your unrealistic expectations, then expect to be obsessed with dieting and preoccupied with your weight for many years to come. Because the alternative to peace is preoccupation.

Weight Wars: Your Vanity vs. Your Sanity

I loved it when one of my clients said, "I don't care what I weigh, I just want to be able to look down and see my feet again." When she uttered those words, I knew she was starting off on the right foot. But she wasn't always this pragmatic and lighthearted about her weight. The birth of her baby dramatically changed the way she felt about her body; it initiated the rebirth of her body acceptance. As she described it, "Looking back, I can't believe that I was so concerned about my looks and preoccupied with my weight. I'd be thinking about how I could lose weight while I was at work, at the movies, driving in the car, exercising at the club, on a dinner date with my girlfriends, at the playground with my niece, even while I was having sex with my husband. My little baby girl has changed all that. When we're together, I want to be there 100 percent, not off somewhere daydreaming about how I can burn more calories. When she asks to play a game, I want to be able to say 'yes' instead of 'no, mommy has to do her exercise.' When she asks to make chocolate chip cookies, I want to say 'great idea' instead of 'no, mommy can't eat cookies; they're too fattening.' Feeling good is now more important than looking good—and it feels great to no longer be a prisoner of dieting."

In the great battle against weight, sometimes we have to choose between feeling good and looking good (at least by society's standards), and oftentimes we have to decide between our sanity and our vanity. If looks, the thin ideal, and a size-six figure drive our thoughts and actions, most likely our sanity will be compromised. We'll wake up every morning at odds with our bodies, refusing to eat in the name of weight loss, and blaming our pregnancy (and sometimes our children) for our weight struggles. The number one reason given by women who don't want to have children is that they don't want to lose their figures. There are many valid reasons not to get pregnant, but in my opinion, vanity shouldn't be one of them. Age and menopause will do a number on your figure anyway. And there is so much more to life than thin thighs.

"What else could there be?" said Lindsay half-jokingly. "Thin thighs are the answer to all of life's problems." She also loved to tell her favorite joke about a woman who finds a magic lantern and a genie appears granting her the one wish of her dreams. Without missing a beat, the woman answers, "I wish for thin thighs!" In light of world problems and environmental decay, the genie begs her to reconsider her selfish wish. "All right then," the woman responds. "Thin thighs for all women in the world!"

All joking aside, thin thighs have clouded our thinking, and a number of national polls have verified that we've lost our perspective when it comes to weight. *Psychology Today* asked whether we would choose to be fifteen pounds thinner or live five years longer. *Glamour* magazine asked if we'd rather have a successful career, a meaningful relationship, or a thin body. Another survey asked if we'd rather have an all-expenses-paid trip around the world, sex with a celebrity, or a 36-24-36 figure. In every case, we chose thinness. What has happened to us? When did a superficial number on a scale supersede meaningful life pursuits such as health, longevity, love, world experiences, and a fling with Tom Cruise? When dieting and the thin ideal took over women's lives back in the 1960s. Since then, the pursuit of thinness has been placed above and beyond all other life pursuits, and it sadly seems "normal" for women to value thinness over love, success, happiness, and a meaningful life.

I wish someone would do a survey asking mothers this question: Would you rather have a perfect size-six figure or more quality time with your children? My guess is that most of us would choose our children over chiseling down to a size six. *We may have lost our perspective, but motherhood can help us gain it back.* Somehow by way of the umbilical cord, we acquire a greater sense of life's purpose and realize that the time it takes to pursue the thin ideal takes precious time away from our children. Studies have found that women spend one third of their waking hours worrying about weight, food, and fat—that's almost six hours of brain space wasted each day. I don't know about you, but I don't have six seconds to waste anymore, never mind six hours. If I did, I'd be playing peekaboo with my little Tyler, reading to him, walking him, and cuddling him. I wouldn't be adding up my fat grams, counting calories, getting on the scale, or grabbing the flab on my stomach with desperation. But given my professional and personal antidieting mission, I chose peace over vanity long ago.

Needless to say, if you forgo peace and opt for weight preoccupation instead, it won't make you a better mother, a sexier partner, or a happier woman. And it won't make you thin. In fact, being obsessed about weight loss prevents weight loss. When you are anxious and uptight about your weight, your fat cells are in constant angst. "Oh boy, here she goes again. She stepped on the scale this morning, cried out some expletives, skipped breakfast, then asked her husband if her butt looked too big. Doesn't he learn? Why can't he just say, 'No honey, you look great'?" Your fat cells respond to your weight preoccupation (and your husband's clueless comments) by shutting down fat release. *But when you relax, your fat cells will relax, too, and when they relax, they release more fat.*

Researchers at Cornell University and elsewhere found that those postpartum women who are less anxious about losing weight, lose more weight and are more likely to get back into their prepregnancy clothes within a year than those who are weight obsessed. It's been proven! *The more relaxed you are about losing weight, the more successful you'll be.*

So relax, save your sanity, and slim down your body at the same time. Being relaxed about your weight doesn't mean putting your feet up with the remote control in one hand and bonbons in the other. Relaxing about your weight isn't a behavior, it's an attitude. An attitude that allows you to be patient, permits imperfection, puts your body in control of your weight-loss schedule, and takes pleasure in eating without fretting about potential weight gain. *An attitude that acknowledges that your baby couldn't care less what you weigh—he or she thinks you're the most beautiful woman in the world, even if you can't fit into your 501s.*

If you've had other children, you've been through this before and hopefully already have a more relaxed attitude, a clearer picture of what to expect, and a better sense of what will keep you sane about your weight. With a toddler running around and/or children to taxi around and/or teenagers gallivanting around, thin thighs and tight abs aren't your biggest concern—time is.

So Many Fat Cells, So Little Time

Time—it's a precious commodity that's in great shortage; the one thing that every mother wants more of. My friends who had their kids years ago used to tell me that they'd sell their soul for a twenty-five-hour day, that they would pray for their baby to sleep just fifteen minutes longer, that the only present they wanted for Mother's Day was time to themselves. After years of pretending to understand, nodding in agreement, and sharing my childless time restraints, I now know exactly what they meant: babies and children cause some kind of permanent glitch in the time continuum.

We look at the clock one minute, it's 9 A.M. We glance at the time the next minute, it's 5 P.M. How did that happen? What did we do in eight hours? I know what I didn't do. I didn't return phone calls, didn't take a shower, didn't make it to the grocery store, didn't pay the bills, and didn't turn on the computer to write. I used to be able to spend an uninterrupted eight hours immersed in my writing. Now, when I turn on the computer, it's a telepathic alarm clock for him. And wouldn't you know it, I hear him downstairs as I'm typing these words.

So, you can now trust me when I tell you that I'm sensitive to your time shortage and sensible about helping you fit the Postpartum Peace Plan into your hectic schedule. When you say, "I just can't do it. I don't have the time" I believe you—and I'll provide realistic solutions that real-life mothers can implement. For example:

- Can't sit down to a small meal? No problem; standing burns more calories anyway.
- Can't cook a meal? Take-out and home-delivered meals work great when there's no cook in the kitchen. And soup and a sandwich work great when there is a cook in the kitchen, but she just doesn't want to cook.
- Can't make it to the grocery store? Have no fear, the Internet is here. Online shopping does save time.
- Can't make it to the 6 A.M. aerobics class? Bring the class to you with a video; there are dozens specifically designed for post-pregnancy.
- Can't make it through the whole sixty-minute video? Go straight to the ab work one day and the cardio portion the next. At least you'll feel that you're doing something.
- Can't find the time to finish reading this book? Don't try to read it all at once; a section or chapter at a time is perfectly fine.

This book and the Postpartum Peace Plan will not rob you of time you don't have. The last thing I want to do is add another stressful time constraint to your already overbooked schedule. A new mother's workload would tire an Olympic athlete and put a workhorse to shame. We are still doing everything we did before having children—the cleaning, shopping, gardening, bill paying, event scheduling, appointment scheduling, financial planning, retirement planning, trip planning—plus an average of ten hours a day of baby care (sounds like an underestimate to me). Then, on top of our already demanding home schedule, two thirds of us go back to work full- or part-time. Working mothers put in eighty-five hours a week between the office and home—that's more than two full-time jobs! In addition to feeling stressed, exhausted, and time-challenged, we also feel guilty for not keeping up like we think we should. We haven't written the thank-you notes, sent out the birth announcements, painted the nursery, joined the mother's group, researched day care, detailed our cars, washed the windows, spring cleaned our house, or revamped our bodies. How could we? There simply are not enough hours in the day.

What Have You Got to Lose?

By following the time-sensitive Postpartum Peace Plan and giving PEACE a chance, the only thing you'll lose is weight—naturally, safely, and permanently. Studies have shown that the weight you lose during the postpartum months is more likely to be maintained than any other weight loss in your life. Unlike the weight you may have lost for your wedding, Caribbean cruise, or high school reunion, you won't gain it back. *This weight loss is for you—and it's forever.*

It doesn't matter if you were underweight or overweight before you got pregnant; if you gained fifteen pounds during your pregnancy or fifty; if this was your first pregnancy or your fifth; if you had twins or triplets; if you had a vaginal birth or C-section; if you are twenty years old or forty years old; if you had your child six days ago or six years ago—the Postpartum Peace Plan is your solution to shape up, slim down, and save your sanity. It will give you the relaxed attitude, the right time line, and the realistic strategies you need to keep both you *and* your fat cells happy.

So what have you got to lose? *Absolutely nothing—except weight.*

Chapter Three

Old Myths About Being a New Mother

After I explained the Postpartum Peace Plan to Jill, she emphatically stated, "It sounds great, and it makes sense, but it won't work for me. At age forty, I added sixty-five pounds to my already overweight frame with twin girls and delivered them with an emergency C-section. I'm unable to breastfeed and it's the dead of winter, so I can't exercise much either. This plan won't work for me; nothing will work for me. I'm doomed to be an overweight mother."

Many women, like Jill, feel doomed from the start, convinced that their bodies, pregnancy experience, and/or after-birth situation are working against their weight loss efforts. But most of what we hear about the difficulties of postpartum weight loss are myths that we erroneously think are true because we've heard them enough times. Our mothers, mothers-in-law, grandmothers, aunts, great-aunts, sisters, friends, masseuses, personal trainers, cosmetologists, psychics, and sometimes even our doctors, pediatricians, nurses, midwives, and nutritionists have told us:

- If you were overweight before getting pregnant, you'll be really overweight after.
- If you're forty or over when you have your first child, you'll struggle with weight forever.
- If you gained more than thirty-five pounds during pregnancy, you'll be overweight after.
- If you had a C-section, you'll never get your weight or waist under control again.
- If you have more than one child, each one will add a ten-pound layer of fat.
- If you have another child too soon, you'll retain more weight.
- If you don't breastfeed, you'll have more difficulty losing the weight.
- If your mother struggled with postpartum weight loss, you will too.
- If you went over term, you'll lose less weight than if you delivered early or on schedule.
- If your baby weighed more than ten pounds, you'll weigh more after birth.
- If you had a girl, you'll lose less weight than if you had a boy.
- If you delivered in winter, you'll hang on to more fat than if you delivered in summer.

All these anxiety-producing, weight-condemning ifs! Let me add one more to this list: If you believe any or all of these myths, then you will have a more difficult time losing the weight. Sooner or later, you'll throw in the towel in defeat, convinced that nothing will work for you because everything is working against you. But as you'll discover in this chapter, there is little, if any, scientific evidence to support these myths. Postpartum weight loss is *not* determined by "old wives' tales," rumors, or half-truths. It's determined in part by gender (by virtue of being women, we are all endowed with stubborn female fat cells), and in part by genetics (by virtue of our genes, some of us have downright obstinate fat cells, but that's true throughout our lives, not just during the postpartum period). But the biggest determining factor of postpartum weight loss is *lifestyle.* By virtue of our behaviors and choices, our postpartum fat cells can either become larger and more powerful than gender and genetics combined, or smaller and more amenable than they've ever been in their lives. *How we structure our lives, our eating, and our activity level is what influences our ability to lose weight after birth.*

As it turned out, Jill was not doomed by her gender or her genetics, and she was not destined to struggle with weight because of her twin girls, sixty-five-pound weight gain, emergency C-section, season of birth, or inability to breastfeed. Instead, she took control of her lifestyle and her weight fate with the Postpartum Peace Plan—and it worked beautifully for her. She not only lost all sixty-five pounds, but another ten that she was unnecessarily carrying around. If the Postpartum Peace Plan worked for Jill, it will work for you, too. Jill's story is just one of the many real-life scenarios I'll share of women who have outsmarted their postpartum fat cells when they never thought they could.

But I Gained Fifty Pounds!

Tara was beside herself with regret. "Why didn't I watch my weight more carefully while I was pregnant? Why didn't I eat less and exercise more? I didn't consciously try to gain this much weight, it just sort of happened, and before I knew it, I looked like a beached whale. Now, I'll never get this weight off. Why didn't my doctor make me limit my weight gain to twenty-five or thirty pounds?"

Because her doctor knew better than to restrict her weight gain, and hopefully yours did, too. Limiting pregnancy weight gain can limit the health of your baby, so your physician should be praised, not blamed. Just be thankful you didn't get pregnant back in the 1950s when obstetricians were prescribing diet pills and putting women on low-calorie food plans to keep their weight gain down to fifteen pounds. Could you imagine gaining only fifteen pounds? My left thigh weighed more than that by my second trimester! It didn't take long for research to discover that this kind of drastic weight restriction compromised the health of both the mother and the baby, so by the 1970s, women were encouraged to gain up to twenty-five pounds (but no more!) to prevent low-birth-weight infants. And thankfully over the last thirty years, we have been given even more leeway with the doctor's scale. Although the Institute of Medicine still recommends a maternal weight gain of twenty-five to thirty-five pounds, most doctors share the philosophy that each woman's body will gain the appropriate amount of weight for her personal situation—and as long as she's not consuming a quart of Häagen-Dazs, a pound of chocolate, a bushel of apples, a side of beef, and a wheel of cheese every day, her weight gain should not be over-scrutinized.

So I asked Tara, "Why do you think you gained fifty pounds during pregnancy?"

1. Did you use pregnancy as an excuse to overeat morning, noon, and night?
2. Did you use pregnancy as a rationale to lie on the couch all day watching soaps?
3. Did you eat well and move your body—and your body just naturally gained fifty pounds?

Tara chose door number three. She ate well, but didn't go nuts on high-sugar, high-fat foods. She walked three times a week, but didn't turn down an opportunity to relax her tired joints and muscles either. Her body seemed to want to gain this amount of weight. And if her body naturally needed to gain fifty pounds, then it would naturally lose fifty pounds (or close to it), too.

"Wait a minute!" Tara argued. "I've been on the Internet doing some research and found some studies that said the more weight you gain during pregnancy, the more weight you'll retain, especially if it was over thirty-five pounds—and I gained almost 50 percent above that!" To be honest, there is some research pointing to what is deemed "excessive weight gain" during pregnancy as the culprit in hindering weight loss after. But none of the studies I've come across looked at women's eating and exercise habits during pregnancy, or their eating and exercise habits after. So, we don't know if they gained a lot of pregnancy weight because they ate a lot of food, or if they retained a lot of postpartum weight because they were still eating a lot of food. In other words, we don't know their *lifestyle*—that number one determining factor of postbaby weight loss. In addition, many of these studies only followed women for three or six months after birth, not nearly enough time for any woman to lose pregnancy weight, and definitely not enough time for those women who gained fifty or sixty pounds. Other, better-designed studies that did follow women for a year or more showed that pregnancy weight gain does *not* affect postpartum weight loss. For example, a recent study at the University of Iceland found that women can reach their prepregnancy weight regardless of gestational weight gain. Those that gained the most weight during pregnancy just took a little longer to lose it.

Tara admitted that she came across this study from Iceland, too, but chose to focus on those that gave her the more "doom and gloom" outlook. "I was looking for something to justify my frustration and give me a reason for my struggle. But if my fifty-pound pregnancy weight gain isn't the reason why I can't lose weight, then what about the fact that I went two weeks over term and delivered an eleven-pound baby in the middle of winter?" Tara had also come across some online information (or should we say misinformation?) pointing to her forty-two weeks of gestation, her winter delivery, and the high birth weight of her baby as explanations for her higher than average postpartum weight. These factors couldn't be used to justify her weight frustration either. *A bigger baby does not lead to a bigger mother, going over term does not undermine weight loss, and season is not a reason for postpartum weight retention.* The truth was that she didn't need any reason for her weight struggle; she was struggling because just about all women do. And she could eventually lose the weight like any other woman as long as she made peace with her fat cells by focusing on her postbaby lifestyle with the Postpartum Peace Plan.

Two of the PEACE principles were most instrumental for Tara's weight turnaround: (1) embracing her body through the many stages of postpartum weight loss, and (2) actively moving it particularly after the third month. By walking three to five times a week (most of the time accompanied by her baby in a backpack), she sped up her weight loss—and by the end of her twelfth month, she was down forty-six pounds and "feeling pretty damn good" about herself. If you gained a lot of weight (or "loads of lard" as Tara called it), please don't waste any time beating yourself up. Instead, beat the pavement and get out there and walk, stroll your baby, or run if that's your thing—just move! And if you gained more than the recommended weight because you ate nonstop for nine months straight without coming up for breath, don't spend any time feeling guilty about it now. Get going and make some changes in your lifestyle. Instead of eating for two, you can learn to eat for *you.*

But I Was Overweight Before I Had Two Kids Thirteen Months Apart!

Mary couldn't remember a day in her adult life when she didn't feel fat. She went on her first diet at age twelve, and since then has barely come up for air, going on and off every diet known to women. As she said, "My fat cells were already huge before I got pregnant for the first time, then four months later we had a little accident, and I didn't have a chance to lose the first pregnancy weight before the scale started creeping up once again. I wanted to wait at least two years between pregnancies, but instead my body was pregnant for almost two years straight. Now the layers of fat from each pregnancy are making me so depressed and embarrassed that I barely leave the house. When I do find the courage to venture out the front door, I make sure my babies are with me so at least people will know why I'm so fat."

Mary had many past and present weight issues weighing her down and needed intensive support, understanding, and education to put her situation in perspective. To begin lightening the load, I spent some time dispelling the "Two-Year Rule" as it's called—waiting at least two years before getting pregnant again so that your body and fat cells have time to fully recover. In reality, this rule is more to protect your brain cells than to help shrink your fat cells—two kids in diapers, two kids wanting their bottles, two kids needing baths, two kids to stroll, carry, console, and put to sleep is enough to make any woman lose a few brain cells. But as far as your fat cells are concerned, the Two-Year Rule doesn't rule. There's little research to prove it, and in fact, a study from the University of Greenwich in London found that the longer the intervals between pregnancies, the more weight women retained. Go figure! There are no tried-and-true facts when it comes to postpartum fat.

Next, I took on the "each child adds ten pounds" myth. It's not necessarily more difficult to lose weight after the second child. A Swedish study found that women generally lose more weight after the second child than after the first. At the beginning, weight loss may be slower after the second pregnancy, but at six months, those fat cells are off and running, shrinking faster than after the first pregnancy. What about after your third, fourth, or fifth child? Unfortunately, minimal research exists to give you an answer, but the third pregnancy may be more difficult, the fourth a bit easier, and the fifth and beyond nobody knows for sure.

Then, I tackled the "overweight before, obese after" myth. Another Swedish study (we can thank the Swedes for the bulk of the research on postpartum weight retention) found that a woman's weight before getting pregnant does not determine her weight after delivery. A woman can be underweight before and overweight after, or a woman can be overweight before and at a normal, comfortable weight after. Pregnancy is a life-changing event in many ways, and one of those ways may be a renewed investment in our health and fitness. During pregnancy, most of us eat healthier than ever before in our lives, and after pregnancy, we want to continue eating this way because it gives us the energy to care for our children as well as the vitality to actively participate in our children's and grandchildren's lives in years to come.

Last, I tackled the real reason Mary was "wrestling with her weight" (she vividly described her fat cells as Sumo wrestlers and herself as Pee Wee Herman)—her years of dieting. Research has found that the greater number of diets you went on before you got pregnant, the greater your weight now—and over six diets appear to really tip the scales in your fat cells' favor. Mary recounted that she'd been on so many diets that she couldn't begin to count, but her guess was "a hell of a lot closer to sixty than six."

Perhaps this is the real underlying reason why most women struggle with postpartum pounds. The typical woman has been on at least fifteen diets, and those previous episodes of self-starvation made our thirty billion fat cells take full advantage of fat storing during pregnancy and then coveting that stored fat during the postpartum period.

The bulk of my work with Mary was to convince her that she could undo the damage of her dieting past and get down to a comfortable weight for the first time in her adult life. All five PEACE principles were vital for her, and by taking care of herself with food, fitness, stress management, and a little pampering—she was soon able to venture confidently out in public without her babies—and eventually was able to take full pride in her forty-pound lighter new, trim body.

But My Mother Was Overweight!

Sue desperately wanted to point the genetic finger of blame at her mother. "My mother gained forty-two pounds with me; I gained exactly forty-two pounds with my daughter. My mother never lost twenty-five of those pounds, and I'll never speak to her again if I stay twenty-five pounds heavier for the rest of my life!" Sue also recalled her mother blaming her for her weight problem. "If she said it once, she said it a thousand times, 'It's because of you that I wear a size eighteen and can't shop in regular department stores.' I always felt responsible for her weight problem."

"So, do you want to do the same thing to your mother and blame her for your weight problem?" I asked. "And do you want to keep passing the blame and make your daughter feel responsible for your weight struggles, too?" She looked up at me sadly and answered, "No. I really don't. I don't want to blame my mother, and I definitely don't want to put my daughter on a guilt trip about my weight. I just want to lose the weight."

And she did. Despite her genetic tendency to have larger fat cells, she took responsibility for her own eating and exercise habits with the Postpartum Peace Plan and lost most of the forty-two pounds without uttering another negative word about her mother.

Genetics can have a powerful effect on how much weight we gain during pregnancy, some effect on how quickly we lose the weight after, but little effect on how much *total weight* we lose. In other words, research has found that your genes can slow down your ability to fit into your prepregnancy jeans, but you *will* eventually fit into them. Your own postpartum behaviors, not your mother's weight, is what will determine how much weight you'll lose. And it was your mother's postpartum behaviors that caused her to be a size eighteen (or any other size) after having you. Ask your mother about her eating and exercise habits in the year following your birth. Was she active? Did she follow some fad diet? Did she do nothing to lose weight?

After asking her mother these questions, Sue discovered that her mother never really did much of anything to lose those last twenty-five pounds. She went on and off a few crazy diets, but she never exercised regularly and she never focused on eating moderately. And Sue summed up the mother–daughter weight connection perfectly, *"You may inherit stubborn fat cells, but you don't inherit behaviors. You choose them. And I'm choosing to lose these last twenty-five pounds with positive eating and exercise behaviors."*

BUT I HAD MY FIRST CHILD AT FORTY!

With the surge of pregnancies for women in their forties, I've had many clients believe that age was working against them, but Jessica's story is one that immediately comes to mind. She first came to see me when she was four months pregnant because she was prematurely worried that her "older, already sagging, less elastic body would stay pregnant looking when she was pregnant no more." She was convinced that her body would be "permanently stuck in the pregnancy position" for the rest of her life.

I quickly put her in touch with other forty-plus-year-old new mothers, who reassured her that her body did have some spring left and could look very "unpregnant" with a little effort. With these women's kind words, her age anxiety started to lift. Then I shared with her some research showing that if older women do lose less weight, it's by choice, not by year of birth. Many older women are less obsessed with thinness (we've been there, done that—and it hasn't done us much good) and accept a postpartum weight that is healthy and vital instead of emaciated and weak. And her anxiety was just about gone when I told her that I, too, was pregnant at forty and due about the same time she was. She was very excited to hear this news, and she came to view me as her postpartum support buddy as well as her nutritionist. As it turned out, her body ended up springing back more quickly than mine, and she was "floating on cloud nine" nine months after delivery.

What helped Jessica the most was this bit of advice: Match your meals to your decade. Whatever decade of life you're in, make sure you eat at least that many meals. This recommendation is based on research at Tufts University that found that our ability to burn off a meal dramatically declines as we grow older. Twenty-year-old women could burn up one thousand calories in one sitting with little effort, while women in their forties could only metabolize four hundred to five hundred calories at one time. What this means is that older new mothers need to eat four to five small meals to lose weight. Jessica was actually thrilled with this news. "I get to eat more often and still lose weight! Life does get better with age."

But I Had Twins with a C-Section!

Hanna was taken by surprise when her ultrasound revealed twins, and then taken by surprise again when her doctor informed her that she had to have a C-section. "Another surprise I didn't need, but I'm absolutely shocked that I'm having such a difficult time losing weight. I've never had a problem with my weight before. Do double the babies mean double the weight retained?"

Hanna was only four weeks postpartum when she made an appointment with me, and I told her, "No, multiple births do not multiply your weight loss difficulties. You can lose just as much weight as you would have with a single birth, but now is not the time, your body is still recovering from birth and cesarean surgery. Go home, give yourself another couple of months to adjust and heal, and then we'll tackle your weight." When she came back at fourteen weeks, she was already feeling much better about her weight prognosis. She had lost almost ten pounds without even trying.

If you had a C-section, you probably weren't happy about it, and left the hospital with a painful, distended stomach filled with gas. But you may be happy to hear that having one has been found to speed up postpartum weight loss in the first few months. A C-section is major surgery that requires energy, calories, protein, and nutrients to heal the incision and recover from the trauma. And as with any abdominal surgery, a C-section also makes it uncomfortable and often painful to eat, so women automatically eat less to ease the discomfort.

As expected, Hanna's postsurgical weight loss came to a halt within a few weeks, and then picked up again when she began following the Postpartum Peace Plan. After about a year, she was feeling at peace with her weight, but was still battling her stomach and waist. "Will I ever have a flat, smooth stomach again?" she asked. With a C-section, the abdominal muscles are cut as well as stretched, and they may never heal back to their original state or be as strong and compact as they were before pregnancy. Hanna wasn't happy with my forthright answer and followed up with a hopeful look. "What about with plastic surgery? Can't I pay for tight, perfect abs?" Tummy tucks, liposuction, and laser surgery can help get rid of the extra skin and obstinate fat, but all the top surgeons of the world can't perfectly reconnect the abdominal muscles to make them tight and toned. She sat there thinking for a moment and replied, "So all the king's horses and all the king's men can't put Hanna's tummy back together again?" It was obvious that she had been singing nursery rhymes to her twin daughters.

Speaking of her daughters, Hanna also asked if it was true that daughters make it harder to lose the weight than sons. No, it's not true that "girls add girth from birth." There is absolutely no proof, scientific or otherwise, that the sex of our children sabotages our weight-loss efforts. So, Hanna embraced her daughters with a hug and embraced her body and her belly with acceptance and admiration for delivering healthy, beautiful twin girls. She had always wished for daughters, and thanked her body for making that wish come true.

But I'm Breastfeeding, Exercising, and Eating Right!

Cathy was a personal trainer who had been in tip-top shape before she got pregnant. She and everyone else thought that her personal and professional investment in health and fitness would guarantee a quick return to her fit and firm form. That was not the case, and at eight months postpartum, she came to see me. "It's so ironic. Here I am helping other people get fit and lose weight, but now I can't seem to help myself—me, of all people—the fitness fanatic! I feel like I'm doing everything right: breastfeeding my baby, eating nutritiously, and exercising. What is wrong with my body?"

Nothing was wrong with Cathy's body. Even though she was a personal trainer, she was still a woman with stubborn postpartum fat cells. And even though she was a fitness fanatic, she was still a breastfeeding mother whose body was protecting its fat stores to provide adequate milk for her baby. But as we spent some time working on patience and realistic expectations, we did discover that something was wrong with her eating. Although she was eating nutritious fruits, vegetables, and whole grains, she wasn't eating enough food—and especially not enough fat. Her diet was mostly vegetarian with little animal or dairy products and almost no fat. And without enough fat and calories in her diet, she couldn't burn fat in her body. When we don't consume at least a serving or two of fat a day, our bodies go into a semistarvation state where metabolism and fat-burning potential slow down. Eating a very-low-fat diet threatened Cathy's fat cells and caused them to put up the weight loss barriers, but after adding some olive oil, avocado, and cheese to her daily diet, she felt those barriers give way and could "feel the fat being released again."

But she still wasn't satisfied with the outcome. She said her body was "twelve terrible pounds away from her petite prepregnancy weight." She didn't look like she needed to lose twelve pounds to me, so I asked what she weighed before she got pregnant, and she quickly answered, "A terrific 120 pounds!" Then I asked her what she weighed at her first prenatal visit, and she told me 130 pounds. "So you gained ten pounds in the first eight weeks of your pregnancy?" and she looked at me without answering.

That was the pivotal question for Cathy. She realized that she had underestimated her prepregnancy weight (a common occurrence for women), which in turn overestimated her postpartum weight. She had been saying that she weighed 120 pounds for the last decade, regardless of what the scale said. Her driver's license verified it, but her driver's license also said that she was a blue-eyed blonde (only her hair dresser and optometrist know for sure) who was an inch taller than reality. What does your driver's license say? That little white weight lie can cause big dark problems when it comes to our perceived goals. If we underestimate our prepregnancy weight, we're setting ourselves up for unattainable goals, weight loss failure, and body disappointment.

After much discussion, Cathy and I concluded that she was not twelve pounds away from her prepregnancy weight, but more like a manageable and acceptable four pounds—and finally she was quite satisfied with the outcome.

But I Had My Baby Four Years Ago!

Betty marched into my office, plopped herself down on the couch, flung her hair back, and brought me to attention. "Listen up, honey. I am in desperate need of your kindly assistance. I never lost the twenty pounds from when I had my dear, sweet Josh four long years ago, and now it pains me to say that I'm a tad bit afraid my chances have come and gone like a groundhog on Groundhog Day. But I figured if anyone could help me, I'd put money on you. This extra weight is really cramping my style on the dance floor. I used to be a two-step state champion in my day, but now I don't have the energy to tear up the dance floor like I used to. So what do you think? Can you help a not-so-new mother in distress?"

It probably goes without saying that Betty was from the South, the "real South" as she called it—Mississippi, to be exact. "Where I come from, sweetheart," she explained, "there are two types of filling stations: one for filling up your car and one for filling up your stomach. And the All-You-Can-Eat-for-$5.95 filling stations are a heck of a lot more popular than the other kind. Hell, we all only fill up our gas tanks so we can get to the all-night diners where there's enough fried chicken, barbecued ribs, corn on the cob, and peach cobbler to feed a small army. Food in the South is food for the soul."

Betty had a major case of what I call "portion distortion." A portion was not a cup or a serving; it was a whole casserole dish, pie tin, or side of ribs. She continued to explain her "fill 'em up" eating philosophy: "My dear passed mother, God rest her soul, taught me two overriding rules in the kitchen. First, always bite off more than you can chew. And second, always double the recipe even if you're the only one eating. I can't break those rules now; she'll strike me dead from the grave. I just know she will."

Unlike the previous story about Cathy, Betty had no problem eating, and she had no problem embracing her body. In her endearing southern drawl, she said, "I don't mind one bit being a larger woman. These melon-sized breasts produced enough milk to feed ten Joshs, and these big hips still carry him around like a charm at forty-five pounds. Not to mention the fact that my husband loves something to grab onto when we're engaged, if you know what I mean. But I just can't live another day being this large; it's hard on the joints and hard on the feet. If you even made me ten pounds lighter, I'd be lighter on my feet on the dance floor, and a very happy woman."

My work with Betty began by giving her a different notion of portions, one that both her and her late mother could accept. She could still eat the whole dish, container, or multiple-person recipe—

just not all at one sitting. The casserole could last a couple of days, and the fried chicken could be eaten for breakfast or lunch the next day. As far as the All-You-Can-Eat diners were concerned, she was happy to hear that she could still frequent those establishments, and she soon realized that one plateful (versus five) could satisfy her southern appetite just fine.

Betty found that it's never too late to lose the postbaby weight. She sent me a picture of herself at a country music festival fully clad in a petticoat and cowboy boots—and her beaming smile said it all. She had reached both her weight goal and her dancing goal. You, too, can lose the weight you gained and regain the energy you lost, and do anything and everything that makes you happy. For Betty, that was dancing the night away. For you, it may be riding a bike with your tyke, playing the bongos, painting a picture, climbing a mountain, or starting your own business. Whatever it is, don't let your weight take away the pleasure of immersing yourself in joyous life activities. Instead, take away the excess pounds and grab on to life.

As you can see by the real-life case studies shared in this chapter, there are as many different pregnancy experiences as there are women. We are each biologically different, and therefore, will have our own unique postpartum experiences. I did some of my own research by surveying over three hundred postpartum women, and found virtually no correlation between weight loss and any postpartum variable (except regular exercise, but more on that later), concluding there is no such thing as a "normal" postbaby weight loss experience.

- Some women who gained the most weight during pregnancy, lost the most weight after.
- Some women who gained the least amount of weight during pregnancy, struggled the most to lose it after.
- Some women lost more weight while breastfeeding; others lost more weight after they stopped breastfeeding.

- Some women lost more weight after their fourth pregnancy than after their first.
- Some forty-year-old women lost more weight than twenty-year-old women.
- Some women who had C-sections lost more weight than those who delivered vaginally.
- Some women who went over-term lost more weight than those who delivered prematurely.
- Some women who delivered daughters in winter lost more weight than those who had sons in summer.

So, I can't tell you that you'll have an easier time losing the weight if you are a twenty-year-old, previously thin triathlete, who gained twenty-five pounds, vaginally delivered a seven-pound boy in July, and breastfed him for over a year. And I can't tell you that you'll have a more difficult time if you were forty, flabby, unfit before pregnancy, gained fifty pounds, delivered a ten-pound baby girl by C-section in December, and breastfed her for a week.

What I can tell you is that if you complicate your postbaby weight loss by subscribing to any myths, half-truths, or negative associations, you *will* sabotage your efforts. On the other hand, if you let go of these "old myths about being a new mother" and firmly believe that you are responsible for your own weight loss outcome—*then your journey into new motherhood and postbaby weight loss will be rewarding, satisfying, and successful.*

So, let's embark on that rewarding, satisfying, and successful journey together with the Postpartum Peace Plan.

Chapter Four

The First Six Weeks: Nurturing Yourself as You're Nurturing Your Baby

I relive those first few weeks over and over in my head. From the very first contraction to the very first sight of his beautiful body, from carefully holding his delicate little head to gently kissing his precious little feet, from watching him sleep all swaddled up in his bassinet to watching his umbilical cord fall off and his adorable belly button appear. This was a magical time, the most beautiful and dreamlike of my life—the cooing, cuddling, kissing, hugging, holding, rocking, bouncing, dancing, singing, breastfeeding—the feeling of being helplessly, hopelessly, head-over-heels in love. I often wish I could go back to those memorable first weeks just so that I could love, care, nurture, and soothe him some more.

But there is someone else in my postpartum memory who also needed love, attention, nurturance, care, soothing, and cuddling. That someone is *me*. If I have time to linger in my newborn memories (which doesn't happen very often these days, now that my son is an active toddler moving a million miles a minute), I also recall the overwhelming fatigue, sleepless nights, incapacitating pain, endless bleeding, breast engorgement, sore nipples, afterbirth contractions, night sweats, and lengthy recovery. And I wish that I could go back to those first few weeks to nurture and soothe myself some more. I needed almost as much care as he did during that magical time, but in retrospect, I realize that I didn't care for myself nearly enough. Few mothers do. When that maternal love, baby euphoria, and new mother bliss kicks in (which is usually immediate and intense), it doesn't even cross our minds that we need rest, sleep, food, water, clothing, and shelter. We exist simply and solely to provide these basic human needs for our babies' survival.

The problem is that we can't exist for very long in baby-on-the-brain mode. The sleep deprivation can become so severe that we nod off while driving (pray our little ones aren't in the car with us at the time). The hunger can become so intense that we fall down the stairs from lightheadedness. The dehydration can become so extreme that we develop a migraine that blurs our vision. The fatigue can become so debilitating that we become disoriented, absentminded, and forgetful. So forgetful and tired, that my husband still has to remind me of how I used to fall asleep just about everywhere and misplace just about everything. I'd nod off while breastfeeding, rocking my baby, talking on the phone, eating dinner, and taking a sitz bath. And if I wasn't falling asleep, I'd forget to take a bath, who I was talking to on the phone, and what I was going to eat for dinner. I can't begin to count the number of times I lost the pacifier, misplaced the Desitin, and couldn't find my breast pads. I truly believe that I would have actually lost a breast if they weren't both firmly attached to my body.

As I have experienced personally and as the research shows inarguably, *when we fail to take care of our own needs during this crucial time, we become less capable of fulfilling the needs of our babies.* Mothers who don't fulfill their need for food can't produce sufficient breast milk; mothers who don't fulfill their need for sleep can't keep their eyes open long enough to rock their babies to sleep; and mothers who don't fulfill their need for rest can't summon the strength to take their babies on their first walk.

The purpose of this important chapter is to help *you* take care of *you,* so that you will have a healthy, speedy recovery, and therefore, be better able to care for your baby. And in case there's any confusion, taking care of you right now does not mean losing weight, burning fat, toning your tummy, or getting back in shape. You may desperately want these body-slimming changes, but they are the last things your body (or your baby for that matter) needs during these first six weeks. Instead your body needs to lose excess fluids, tone its pelvic floor muscles (the stretched out muscles surrounding your vagina), get its uterus back in shape, regain strength, and repair torn tissue. You just went through the most physically challenging event of your life. *Your body needs to recover, and you need to help it recover.*

Those hours you just spent in the hospital, birthing center, or at home with a midwife may have been a labor of love that you don't regret for one nanosecond, but the miracle of birth is real-life, hard labor that takes an amazing toll on the female body.

They Don't Call It Labor for Nothing

The dictionary defines "labor" as "demanding bodily work requiring strength and patience." It's an accurate description, but it doesn't quite do our birth labor justice. Your great-grandfather may have labored in the mines, blasting tunnels through mountains. Your grandfather may have "walked ten miles to work at the docks every day, hauling hundreds of pounds of fish in the pouring rain," as he's repeatedly told you. Your father may have "started working at age eight delivering newspapers at 5 A.M. every morning," as he has also repeatedly informed you. But their "labor" pales by comparison. You just did the equivalent of walking three thousand miles in a day and delivered a seven-plus pound baby through your one-inch tunnel of life. Now that's what I call labor!

Every woman is eager to share her own labor-room story that highlights her strength, patience, and pain resiliency. I'll save you the gory details of my story, but my pelvic bone created a major road-block for hours, I threw up on my husband, urinated on my doctor, shouted obscenities at my nurse (they are truly angels for what they withstand in the labor room), kissed my anesthesiologist, and then immediately blocked out every painful contraction and embarrassing behavior once I set eyes on his beautiful cone-shaped head and counted his fingers and toes.

Sometimes memory loss is a good thing. We remember the joy and forget the pain. Are you already starting to forget? Are you saying things like "it really wasn't that bad" or "the funniest thing that happened was . . ."? As with my story, eventually everyone's labor experience is retold with humor. We want to smile at the beautiful memory, even though we may have been crying through most of the transition and delivery. If we really want to be reminded of the painful specifics, we can always pull out the video or the photos. My sister-in-law was my birth photographer, a task she excitedly volunteered for. During labor, I had a vague recollection of the lightbulb flashing, but was too out of it to know exactly where she was pointing the camera. Two days later, she presented me with a dainty little photo album whose floral print foretold feminine beauty inside. But when I opened it, I cried out in disbelief at the pain on my face and the size of my thighs (most of which could not be attributed to a bad camera angle). As I flipped though the pages, I came to a close-up aerial shot of my nether region and said, "There he is, crowning with his full head of hair," only to be quickly corrected: "No, that was right before he crowned. That's all you, not his hairy head."

Perhaps it's too soon for you to find the humor in your labor experience. The endless pushing, hours of excruciating pain, and perhaps fetal distress, fetal monitors, oxygen masks, and emergency C-sections are still in the forefront of your memory. Maybe, like Suzanne, you feel more guilt than giggles. Instead of a Madonna-like, au naturel delivery using perfect Lamaze breathing every step of the way, she "screamed like a banshee, swore like a comedian on HBO, sweated like a pig, simply forgot everything she learned in Lamaze, and grabbed her doctor by the shirt collar demanding, 'Give me drugs, NOW!' " She felt guilty about giving in to drugs and having an episiotomy—feelings that prevented her from reliving her birth experience with joy.

Perhaps your birth plan didn't quite go according to plan (whose does?), and you had an episiotomy, epidural, other pain medication, or emergency C-section. Does it really matter now? You made it through labor and delivered a beautiful baby. *How you did it is inconsequential; the fact that you did it is monumental.* But I know many women who regret "giving up and giving in to drugs" when they should be rejoicing in their accomplishment. I had an epidural, and I don't feel a twinge of guilt about it. Neither should you if you had one. Relieving pain is not giving up; it enables you to move forward. Asking for drugs doesn't make you weak; it makes you strong enough to deliver your baby into this world. In fact, drug-assisted delivery dates back to biblical times when medicine women gave potent mind-altering herbs to birthing mothers in need. Thousands of years ago, these wise women knew that a mother writhing in pain could not concentrate on the pushing necessary for a healthy birth.

Whatever your course of labor—drugs or no drugs, episiotomy, or C-section—the average woman has three hundred uterine contractions, three thousand muscle contractions, and burns thirty thousand calories during the painful ordeal of birth. And when it's over, your body shows the effort you gave and the pain you endured. You may have broken blood vessels in your eyes and cheeks, dark circles under your eyes, cracked bleeding lips, sore ribs from the breathing and pushing—and that's just from the waist up. The casualties of labor below the belt are even more severe. If you had back labor, you may have a bruised tailbone that can take months to heal. If you had a vaginal birth, all I can say is three words—ice, ice, ice. The tearing, stitches, swelling, hemorrhoids, and bleeding make it difficult to lie down, never mind sit down. If you had a C-section, the gas pains, abdominal bloatedness, deep incision, and layers of stitches through your uterus, muscles, and skin can prohibit you from doing most anything in the first few weeks, from walking up and down stairs to driving a car to dancing with your newborn in your arms.

Regardless of what happened during your birth experience, no doubt you're relieved that it's over. But don't crack open that champagne yet—it's not quite over. Pat yourself on the back for making it through the first two stages of birth: labor and delivery, but save the champagne for when you've completed the important third stage: recovery. And in my opinion, the body's ability to recover from birth is almost as miraculous as birth itself.

Blood, Sweat, and Tears

Over the next six weeks, your female body will undergo a mind-boggling level of recovery. Your uterus will deflate from the size of a beach ball down to a baseball, shrinking ten sizes in forty-two short days. Your blood volume will go back to normal, losing the two extra quarts that it accumulated during your pregnancy. Your perineal tear (or cut if you had an episiotomy) will repair itself, and/or your C-section incision will almost completely heal. Your organs that were pushed, nudged, and shoved for nine months to make room for your growing baby will realign themselves, going back to their proper places in your abdomen. Your diaphragm and liver will descend, your lungs will expand, your pancreas will move back toward center, your bladder will move forward, and your colon will move back up. Everything naturally and miraculously goes back to its original location, shape, and size. Well, almost everything. Your fat cells, muscle tone, and skin elasticity are another story. They take time and effort to get back to their prepregnancy form, and the first six weeks are not the time to put in the effort. *Your body has to recover on the inside before it will reshape on the outside.*

Picture the inside of your body with your uterus being the center of activity during labor and your reproductive organs sustaining the most trauma during delivery. Your body's first healing efforts will be directed to shrinking your uterus, pinching off the placental blood supply, and reconnecting torn tissue in your cervix, birth canal, and perineum. Next, your body will focus outward on your other organs, moving them back to their proper homes. Then, your body will concentrate its efforts on rebalancing your blood volume and body fluids. It's a preprogrammed sequence of life-sustaining healing events that occurs from the inside out. If your body wasn't programmed to heal this way, you could hemorrhage, go into respiratory distress, or have a heart attack from an electrolyte imbalance. Personally, I'm grateful that my body instinctively knows to heal from the inside out. Aren't you?

"Yes and no," replied one of my clients, Darlene. "Of course I want to shrink my uterus and decrease my body fluids, but I also want to shrink my fat cells and decrease my weight, too. It's been three weeks since I've had my baby, but yesterday someone asked me when the baby was due! I burst out into tears right there on the spot, and was so devastated I turned and walked away without even answering." While your body is healing on the inside, don't be surprised if you still look pregnant on the outside; are asked if you're pregnant by people you don't know (and who have no business asking in the first place); or are even still wearing your maternity clothes. It's supposed to be this way. The stretched muscles, loose skin, and inflated fat cells are not life-threatening, and therefore, will be the last to recover. When you know these facts up front, you'll have a better understanding of your body's healing process and won't be taken by surprise when a large, squishy stomach jumps out and scares you half to death.

In fact, I don't want you to be startled or thrown off kilter by any "surprises" during this six-week recovery period. I'm the type of person who doesn't like surprises; I like to know what's going to happen up front so that I can adequately prepare myself. As a health professional, I thought I had a good sense of the biological process of pregnancy and the recovery period. But what I experienced didn't come close to the textbook descriptions of recovery—and it shocked me! To spare you the shock and help prepare you for the reality, here's my wish list for what I wish I knew about the early postpartum period.

- I wish I knew that the bleeding would be more like the Old Faithful geyser than "a heavy menstrual flow." Menstrual flow lasts for four to five days, not four to five weeks, and "heavy" to me means five pad changes a day, not fifteen. "Discharge" is what most of the books call the afterbirth bleeding, but I think "dam-broke" would be a better term. And "lochia" is what the medical folk call it, but I believe Loch Ness Monster would be a more accurate description of what is shed from your body when the uterine lining makes its way out.

- I wish I knew to load my freezer with bags of frozen peas. They are the perfect fit and the perfect temperature for relief between the legs. I also wish I was privy to the idea of putting sanitary napkins in the freezer. Guests may have gasped as they were reaching for some ice, but my torn and stitched perineum would have thanked me.

- I wish I knew that the "after cramps" would rival the intensity of some of my contractions. Like the aftershocks from an earthquake, they can reach high on the Richter scale and send you doubled over on the floor.

- I wish I knew that my first bowel movement would make me think that I was really pregnant with twins but no one knew, and the second one was on its way.

- I wish I knew that night sweats would cause three pajama changes per night, and give me great empathy for all of my menopausal friends.

- I wish I knew to put a mattress protector on my bed—between the "discharge" and the night sweats, it will never be the same.

- I wish I knew how anxious I would be when my baby cried, and how hopeless I would feel when I couldn't do anything to stop it.

- I wish I knew how complicated and painful breastfeeding would be, and what a lifesaver a breastfeeding consultant could be—I would have consulted one right away. Breastfeeding may be natural, but it doesn't always come naturally.

- I wish I knew how absentminded and forgetful I would become and that I would wander from room to room, wondering why I was there, where I meant to go instead, and what I was going to do once I got there.

- I wish I knew that my brain would turn to mush and that I would lose the ability to think, reason, and form complete sentences. MRI scans have recently discovered why our brains seem to go off-line during baby time; they shrink during the last month of pregnancy and don't plump up again for another three months. Presumably, this brain shrinkage is for the welfare of our babies. If we can't focus on anything else, we'll direct all of our mental energy to our newborns.

- I wish I knew that I'd never get more than two hours of sleep at one time. I would have slept more in my last trimester, banking away the extra hours of slumber.

- I wish I knew that maternity leave was really maternity stay: first you don't leave the house at all, then you don't leave without much lengthy planning and preparation with the diaper bag, stroller, car seat, baby carrier, burp cloths, rattles, breast pads, changing pads, and extra changes of clothing for both of us.

Why doesn't anyone tell us these things? Maybe it's because everyone was so busy helping us with infant care that they forgot to mention some important facts regarding postpartum care. Or maybe it's because everyone was trying to protect us with the "what they don't know can't hurt them" philosophy, thinking that fewer women would have children if they knew the whole postpartum truth. We deserve more credit than that. We'd still have children; we'd just be more realistic with our expectations and recovery. We would anticipate these postpartum realities and accept them accordingly, while doing what we could to minimize them.

"I have a wish to add—" volunteered my sister, Lori, who was voted "biggest belly ever" for three straight pregnancies. "I wish I knew that I should never, under any circumstances, get on all fours and let gravity have its way with my stomach." Not only is your stomach lumpy and squishy—it's loose. Pregnancy fooled us into thinking that the belly was taut, tight, and hard. Now that your baby is no longer there to take up the slack, your stretched skin and muscles (not to mention your full, sagging breasts) may hit the floor and send you into a spiral of depression.

Which brings me to my final and perhaps most important wish to share with you—*I wish I knew that postpartum depression doesn't always hit in the first month, but can surface any time in the first year.* I would have prepared myself to be on the lookout for the signs and symptoms well past the first few weeks. As it turned out, I thought I had somehow miraculously bypassed the "baby blues." Having experienced mega-PMS every month, I fully expected to be emotionally paralyzed by dropping postpartum hormones. But as the weeks flew by, my good mood didn't miss a beat. I was happy as a lark, adjusting well, and enjoying my new life as a mother. Then eight months later, my son abruptly stopped breastfeeding, and I stopped dead in my tracks with sadness, loneliness, and confusion.

When it happened, the "baby blues" didn't even cross my mind. My son was crawling, my body was recovered, and my hormones would have surely rebalanced by now. Then I read an article on post-breastfeeding depression, and the biological explanation of my sadness surfaced. Hormones drop again after we stop lactating, especially the hormone oxytocin, which is a mood-elevating hormone that also triggers a boost in brain endorphin and serotonin levels. Endorphins, as you may know, produce a natural high, and serotonin gives a feeling of calmness and serenity. So there it was in black and white—*the boob was good for my mood.* Without the oxytocin, serotonin, and endorphin release, I was going through breastfeeding/brain chemical withdrawal. The feel-good endorphins and antistress serotonin were in short supply, and my brain wasn't at all happy about it.

But withdrawal from breastfeeding wasn't the only cause of my depressed mood. I was also feeling withdrawn from my community, my friends, my family, and my husband. Most of my world was confined to the four walls of my house; my friends had their kids years ago and were busy with their older children or with their careers; my husband was working seventy-five hours a week for an Internet company; and my mother and sister were three thousand miles away in Maine. I felt very much alone and isolated. You may be thinking that the solution to my sadness was obvious—it was time for me to go back to work. But I was working, and had been for some months writing this book and finishing up another one. Every minute my son was napping, I was researching. Every night went he went to sleep and I turned off his light, I went into my home office and turned on my computer. I was home alone with my baby, home alone with my writing, and home alone with my depression. I needed out. I needed companionship, outside stimulation, time away from home, and time with my friends, family, husband, and other new mothers.

As with my situation, postpartum depression is usually caused by a combination of hormonal changes and life changes. The hormonal changes are straightforward and easy to understand. In the few weeks following delivery, estrogen levels plummet and serotonin levels drop with them. Or, as with me, in the few weeks following weaning, oxytocin levels drop, and both serotonin and the endorphins follow suit. The life changes, however, are a bit more complicated and individualized. Having a baby changes your life forever, and some of those changes may cause anxiety, apprehension, and internal conflict. For example, you may feel a shift in your relationship with your partner, family, and friends; you may long for your old, carefree life and your old, cellulite-free body; you may be in conflict about going back to work or staying at home; or you may question your mothering instinct and your decision to even have a child in the first place. These feelings, conflicts, and questions don't make you a bad mother—they make you a healthy, adjusting mother who needs to give herself some time to work out these and other issues and find peace in her new life role.

Thankfully, postpartum depression is finally being talked about more openly in doctor's offices, in women's groups, on talk shows, in Internet chatrooms, and in the popular press. It's about time. Postpartum depression is not new, and it's not rare. Medical documentation dates back centuries, and recent studies have found that 80–90 percent of all new mothers experience some or all of the criteria for depression. That's over three million women each year! A far greater number than those afflicted with any other mental or physical ailment. Of those three million women, about 10 percent will be clinically diagnosed with postpartum depression when their symptoms last more than a few weeks, and 0.1 percent will be diagnosed with postpartum psychosis, a serious condition where hallucinations, delusional thoughts, and irrational behavior can negatively interfere with their babies' care.

Whether you're feeling blue, sad, or downright depressed, you need to know that it's real, normal, and treatable. A study from the National Institute of Mental Health took a random sample of postpartum women and found that 9.3 percent could be clinically diagnosed with depression. Since most women generally do not seek out help for postpartum depression on their own, screening is warranted and necessary so that women can be given the proper therapeutic support and/or drug treatment to make it through the hormonal changes and lifestyle adjustment. If you are feeling sad, hopeless, helpless, confused, out of control, and/or experiencing a lack of interest in everything including your baby, talk to your doctor, midwife, therapist, mother, sister, partner, and friends—*and get the screening and the help you need.*

For the majority of you, however, the baby blues will be a short-lived, normal part of your postpartum recovery, and your sadness will heal just like the rest of your body. As your body recovers from the inside out, the "blood, sweat, and tears" will eventually stop. When your uterus heals, the bleeding will go away (at least until you start your period again). When your body fluids rebalance, the night sweats will disappear (at least until you enter perimenopause). And when your hormones readjust, the tears will dry up (at least until your first PMS attack). Your body will heal itself, unless, of course, you do something that will interfere with its programmed healing process. That something is *dieting.*

DON'T EVEN THINK ABOUT DIETING

Don't let that word enter into your mind or cross your lips. Don't let it start negatively influencing your attitudes and behaviors. Don't let it slow down your postpartum recovery. Don't let it interfere with your future postpartum weight loss. Because it inevitably will. It will cause you to restrict your eating, skip meals, and undernourish your body. It will make you become weight-preoccupied and obsessed with the scale. It will hinder your breast milk production and your body's recovery. And it will cause you to become a fatter postpartum woman with a poorer body image.

As you know from the first three chapters, the D-word (I'm trying to help you not think of it) threatens your fat cells, causes them to protect their stored pregnancy fat, and prevents weight loss. *What you do in the first six weeks determines the speed and success of your weight loss for the rest of the year.* If you cut calories, skip meals, banish bread, forbid sugar, or count grams of fat, your fat cells will deem it unsafe to release fat for months to come. Remember: Your postpartum fat cells are worried about a potential famine. Dieting will only confirm their fears—and they will hold on to their precious stored calories for your survival.

So please take my word for it and don't even think about taking a pill, buying prepackaged foods, or sipping a drink. Because just thinking about doing these things may be enough to cause you to overeat and sabotage your efforts. The University of Washington recently did an interesting study splicing weight loss commercials into a movie. Those women who watched the movie with the weight loss commercials ate hundreds of calories right then and there, while those who watched the movie without the commercials barely ate a thing. If just being reminded of dieting can make you eat more food and eventually gain more weight, imagine what the actual act of restriction will do to your eating. Another study found this out when they put dieting women alone in a room full of cookies for a taste test. One would think that a "taste test" would require just that—a leisurely taste or two to determine the flavor. But these women devoured dozens of cookies in a hurried frenzy. It's been proven: *Dieting doesn't help you eat less; it makes you eat more.*

But at this time in our lives, the dieting–overeating relationship may be the least of our worries. While we need to be gaining strength for recovery, dieting will make us weak, lethargic, disoriented, depressed, and unable to recover from the trauma of birth. And the earlier you start depriving your body of fuel and nutrients, the more devastating the outcome will be. Myra started dieting the second her first contraction hit. "I knew I wouldn't be able to eat anything during labor, so I thought it was a perfect opportunity to fast my way to weight loss. I was actually happy that my labor lasted twenty-eight hours—that was more than a day without eating. Then, I didn't eat anything but fruit for the next two days in the hospital (the food really wasn't worth eating anyway). When I came home, I just kept living on fruit and vegetables for the next month, until I discovered that I wasn't living very well at all. My milk started drying up, my hair was falling out in clumps, and I was so weak that I could barely stand up without feeling like I was going to faint. Then one day, I did faint. I was home alone with my baby and thank God she was sleeping at the time. But I could have been holding her, or something could have happened to her when I was out cold."

Myra's devastating dieting experience may be extreme, but the same could happen to any of you to some degree. If you restrict your eating, you could become malnourished, exhausted, dehydrated, dizzy, and unable to produce breast milk. And you could end up back in the hospital like Myra did. She needed two days of intravenous fluids to rehydrate her body and stabilize her vital signs. But dieting isn't just potentially devastating to your health, it can also have negative effects on your baby. Years ago, I started giving a class to new mothers, warning them of the dangers of dieting by speaking to them from their baby's perspective. I called it, "Mommy, Please Don't Diet," and here are the ten motivating reasons I used to explain why your baby doesn't want you to diet:

1. It makes you too tired to play with me.
2. It makes you too sad to laugh with me.
3. It makes you too weak to carry me.
4. It makes you angry when I want you to be happy.
5. It makes your milk come out too slowly.
6. It makes your milk taste funny. (Dieting can release ketones, a starvation by-product, into your breast milk.)
7. It makes you think about food when you could be thinking of me.
8. It makes you feel ugly when I think you're beautiful.
9. It makes you cover up your body when I want to see it.
10. It makes you sometimes wish that you never got pregnant, when I am always so happy you did.

All very powerful statements, especially number ten. If you haven't blamed your weight struggles on your pregnancy yet, that statement will eventually escape your lips. Or maybe it won't, now that you've read "Mommy, Please Don't Diet," and hopefully you won't diet either. If your baby could talk and say these things wouldn't you walk away from diets forever? We might not avoid the temptation to diet for our own health, but we'd do it (and anything else for that matter) for our babies.

So, if you're not supposed to think about dieting or losing weight, what should you be thinking about during these important first six weeks? Nourishing your body and eating basically the same way you did during pregnancy. This advice holds true whether or not you're breastfeeding. You need ample calories, vitamins, minerals, protein, carbohydrates, fat, and water for a speedy, successful recovery. You need to keep taking your prenatal supplements, and you need to keep eating just as much and just as healthfully as you did for the nine-month growth of your baby.

Most women don't. According to national nutrition surveys, we're coming up short by six hundred to nine hundred calories a day during the postpartum months. That's a lot of calories and a lot of nutrients in those calories that our bodies aren't getting. We erroneously think that we can go back to our old restrictive eating habits once we've delivered a healthy baby. We can't—we need to eat. *Your healthy eating during pregnancy may have ensured a healthy baby, but your healthy eating during the postpartum weeks will ensure a healthy mother.*

Your body is nutritionally depleted from the nine months of pregnancy and from the more recent labor-intensive hours of delivery. This is your replenishing time, and your body can't fully recover if you're not covering all the bases for nutritional adequacy. The same nutrients that were important during pregnancy are equally important during recovery:

- **Folic acid.** It helped form your baby's brain and spinal cord, and it will help your postpartum brain to function more efficiently. Folic acid has been found to reduce depression and increase thinking ability.

- **Calcium.** It helped develop your baby's bones, heart, muscle, and nervous system, and it will help your postpartum bones stay strong as well as calm your mood and improve the quality of your breast milk.

- **Iron.** It helped form your baby's blood supply, and it will help your postpartum red blood cells deliver oxygen to your healing tissue.

- **Vitamin C.** It helped develop your baby's bones, teeth, and wound healing ability, and it will help your postpartum wound healing (or womb healing as I often call it) and tissue repair.

- **Protein.** It helped maximize your baby's muscle mass and birth weight, and it will help you replenish lost muscle and repair any cuts or tears.

- **Carbohydrate.** It helped provide all the energy and B vitamins for the growth of your baby's cells and tissues, and it will help give you the energy to care for your baby and recover from labor. (If it's high in fiber, it will also play the important role of aiding in constipation.)

- **Fat.** It helped form your baby's brain and hormonal system, and it will help your postpartum hormones rebalance. You need fat in your diet to make estrogen in your body.

- **Water.** It enabled all the chemical reactions to occur for your baby's growth, and it will help your postpartum-breast-milk production and kidney function.

These are just a sampling of the nutrients your postpartum body needs for a healthy recovery. In essence, you need every nutrient every day. So don't change a thing with your eating. If anything, up your intake of fresh fruits and vegetables to get some extra nutrients for recovery and breastfeeding. *Don't think less food; think more nutrients.*

EXERCISE YOUR RIGHT NOT TO EXERCISE

While you're not thinking about dieting, you might as well not think about exercising either—at least not in the traditional sense. Not going to the club, not signing up for a kickboxing class, not rejoining your walking group, and not hopping on the stationary bike or stair climber. In fact, I strongly recommend that you exercise your right *not* to exercise during this time. Your body isn't ready, and neither are you. You need to be at home nesting with your newborn, not out pounding the pavement. Your body needs to be in a reclining position for recovery, not in a starting position for a fat-burning race.

"But almost every book and magazine article I've read says that you can start exercising twenty-four to seventy-two hours after giving birth," argued my friend Jackie when we were discussing exercise a week after she gave birth. "I haven't even done one sit-up yet or watched the postpartum exercise video I bought. I feel like I'm late getting started, and I have to get this weight off!" Late? It was still way too soon for sit-ups or aerobics. She should only be lying down on the floor to take a nap and only turning on her VCR to watch a movie—preferably a tearjerker to fulfill the need for a good postpartum cry. Think about how you felt the day after you gave birth: Could you have exercised? I couldn't even get out of bed without feeling like I was ripping from my belly button to my tailbone. The oft-given recommendation to start exercising on day two is not really exercise; it's more like physical therapy. The only "exercises" that are encouraged in the first few days and even weeks are short walks, tummy sucks, and Kegel exercises to increase your blood circulation and aid in your recovery.

"I know what short walks are, but quick, tell me about the tummy sucks and Kegel exercises," asked Jackie, who was desperate to start doing any exercise and was surprised that her doctor hadn't told her about the importance of sucking in her tummy and doing her Kegels. Tummy sucks help to push the uterus back into place, as well as heal and strengthen those stretched out abdominal muscles. Lying down with your knees bent and feet flat on the floor, take a deep breath in and watch your abdomen rise, then as you exhale, suck in your belly button as if you were trying to make it touch your spinal column. Quite simply, that's why they are called tummy sucks. If you'd rather sit than lie down, another variation is what Debbie Herlax, a friend and personal trainer, calls "blow out the candle." Sitting upright in a chair with your weight evenly distributed on both sit bones, inhale through your nose or mouth, purse your lips, and suck in your lower belly as you exhale like you were blowing out a candle.

Now, let's talk about Kegel exercises. They are designed to strengthen and heal another area of stretched out muscles—those of your pelvic floor between your vagina and anus—and are vital if you ever want to sneeze, cough, laugh, or jump without peeing your pants again. The best place to do them is lying in bed, but you can do them while breastfeeding, watching TV, talking on the phone, surfing the Internet, driving in the car, or any other relaxed sitting or lying-down position. All you need to do is firmly tighten the muscles of your pelvic floor by squeezing in your anus and vagina. Hold for eight to ten seconds, or as long as you can, then relax and repeat, working up to twenty-five repetitions four times a day. If you think your Kegels don't need strengthening, test them while urinating. See if you can stop the flow of urine by tightening these muscles. If you can't, then you need to keep doing your Kegels. (An added plus to keep you doing them is that they will also lead to better orgasms—once you're ready to venture into that territory again.)

After doing her tummy sucks and Kegel exercises for a few days, Jackie was still anxious to do "real" exercise and asked, "When can I start doing crunches?" For most women, not for at least a month to six weeks. It takes that long for your diastasis to heal. What is a diastasis? The separation of your abdominal muscles caused from pregnancy. As your baby grew, a gap formed down the center of your stomach as the two sides of your abdominal muscles pulled away. Don't even bother checking for your diastasis the first couple of weeks. I guarantee you it's there. In your third or fourth week, lie on the floor with your knees bent and your feet flat on the ground. Place your fingers below your belly button with your fingertips pointing toward your feet. Slowly lift your head up off the floor and feel for a soft lump protruding from the gap between your muscles. If the gap is greater than two finger widths, slowly put your head back down on the floor, roll over, and carefully get up. Your stomach is not ready for crunches yet, and they may delay your recovery—keep doing your tummy sucks; they will help to close your diastasis. But, if the gap is less than two finger widths, you can start with one or two crunches (see page 156 for instruction) and slowly increase the number as the gap gets smaller.

After a few more weeks of checking her diastasis and finally being able to start doing a few crunches, Jackie asked her final exercise question: "When can I start my cardiovascular, fat-burning aerobic exercises again?" Jackie was disappointed to hear my answer—not until after her OB gives her the okay at her six-week checkup. Exercising too soon can cause increased vaginal bleeding and decreased healing. It can also increase your chances of injury. Your center of gravity is very different now than a few weeks ago when you had a beach ball strapped to your midsection and couldn't bend down to tie your shoes. It takes time to adjust to your new center of gravity and regain your balance. And for some sports, it takes a lot of time—four or more months may be necessary for quick movement activities like tennis, skiing, and step classes.

I'll help you to slowly get into fat burning exercises in the next two chapters, but just in case you think exercise caution doesn't apply to you, you absolutely should not exercise aerobically until you've stopped bleeding; ride a bike until your perineal tear or episiotomy has healed; or do any twisting, jumping, or lifting (nothing heavier than your baby that is) until your C-section has completely healed.

Even if for some reason you get the go-ahead to start exercising aerobically before your six-week checkup, don't expect to burn away your pregnancy fat. Your fat cells are in hibernation and won't cooperate. After how hard they worked to store fat for the nine months of pregnancy, they deserve to be resting, reveling in their glory of ensuring a successful pregnancy and birth.

I'm not saying that you won't lose any weight in the first six weeks. You'll lose enough of weight to keep you happy. You just won't be losing any significant fat weight. You'll lose about five pounds of fluid and blood. And if you add that to the twelve pounds you lost on the delivery table—*you'll lose a total of seventeen pounds or an average of about three pounds a week for the first six weeks!* Not bad by anyone's standards. Your body will get smaller and your maternity clothes will get looser. Remind yourself that you have already lost a great deal of weight, realize that fat loss will soon follow, and don't lose any sleep over your stubborn fat cells. You can't afford to.

When Nobody Sleeps Like a Baby

The bags under your eyes are bigger than the bags of free stuff you brought home from the hospital; your eyes are more bloodshot than a fighter after eight rounds; and your lids are heavier than the infant car seat you're lugging around (I was surprised by its weight!). Sure, you've been sleep-deprived before: in college, when you pulled all-nighters during final exams; at work, when an important report or presentation had to be done; while traveling, when you've crossed numerous time zones with air traffic delays. But in retrospect, these were nothing compared to the chronic, relentless sleep deprivation you're experiencing right now. And I'm sorry to inform you that it's going to get a lot worse before it gets better.

Sleep deprivation is cumulative. Over the next twelve months, you'll accumulate over five hundred hours of sleep debt—the equivalent of almost twenty-one days of total insomnia. Except, of course, that you don't have insomnia. You could close your eyes right now, drift off into dreamland within seconds, and stay there for a thousand years—if, of course, your baby wasn't waking you up every hour or two to feed (they're used to twenty-four-hour womb service!), and if your night sweats weren't waking you up when your baby was in a sound, satisfied slumber.

Your little angel from heaven is a sleep robber. His or her biological rhythms are topsy-turvy, upside down, and flip-flopped. He's just spent the last nine months sleeping during the day (your movement rocked him to sleep) and up most of the night (you probably remember his kicks and jabs in the wee hours of the morning). It can take months for his biological rhythms to right themselves, but you can't wait months to catch up on your sleep. You need it now.

The typical new mother gets only five hours of sleep a night. You may think that's not too bad, you've survived on less before. But during those five hours, we're constantly waking up because we hear our babies, we think we hear them, or our full, painful breasts are begging us to hear them. So, not only do we sleep less, we sleep less soundly with more frequent awakenings. Most of those five hours are spent in stages two and three of sleep where we are easily aroused by our babies' cries for food and comfort. We seldom reach stage four (deep sleep) or stage five (dream sleep) because we're never asleep long enough to get there, and we may never hear our babies if we did. But these deep-sleep stages are vital for our physical and psychological health. Without them, we feel physically depleted and mentally challenged.

"Now that explains a lot," commented my worn-out client, Tanya, who had her first baby five weeks ago. "Yesterday, I practically crawled from room to room searching for my sunglasses so I could go to the store. After three complete house searches, I was so tired that I gave up. When we finally got all buckled up in the car, I tilted the rearview mirror to put on some lipstick—and there they were sitting on the top of my head! And if you think that's bad, wait until you hear what I did this morning. In a semiconscious state, I put toothpaste on my daughter's diaper-rashed bottom and almost brushed my teeth with Desitin!" After we had a really good laugh at her expense, we both concluded that she desperately needed a good night's sleep.

"But how am I going to get it?" demanded Tanya. "My baby girl is up every hour on the hour wanting to feed, and my husband isn't Bessie the Cow so he can't help out in the dairy department." Tanya thought that the only time to sleep was at night, and therefore, the only way to get sleep was to somehow find a way to get her baby to start sleeping through the night. She sought the advice of countless books, websites, and other new mothers. Not surprisingly, nothing worked. What works for one child almost never works for another, it's one of those unsolved mysteries of motherhood. So, instead of wasting any more precious potential sleep time waiting for her baby to start sleeping through the night (which may not happen for a year or more in some unfortunate cases), I informed Tanya that it's almost always easier to sleep when her baby sleeps.

Newborns may be up much of the night, but they're sleeping most of the day—which at least gives us ample opportunity to catch up on some lost sleep, if we only took advantage of it. While they're down for one of their numerous naps, we're up returning phone calls, opening gifts, writing thank-you notes, sending out birth announcements, reading our newborn books, cleaning the house, or simply staring at them lovingly while they're getting their much-needed sleep. Up until relatively recently in history, mothers and babies around the world could be found napping side by side any time of the day. But somewhere in the last century, the modern, industrialized work ethic changed all that, and today, few mothers give themselves permission to nap.

"There's no way I can nap," protested Tanya. "The phone doesn't stop ringing, someone's at the door every thirty minutes to drop off food or a gift, and I have a million things to catch up on while she's napping." Tanya's protests were replaced with possibilities when she used the following five sleep strategies to make her lifestyle more conducive and permissive to daytime napping:

1. Turn off the phone ringer and let your personal secretary, your answering machine, take your calls. Just be sure to turn down the volume so you won't be tempted to listen for who it is.
2. Disconnect the doorbell and put a sign on the door that reads MOTHER AND CHILD SLEEPING, PLEASE COME BACK LATER.
3. Stay in your pajamas all day so that you'll be ready to crawl under the covers at every opportunity.
4. Choose at least one napping time during the day and make it a mother-and-child siesta.
5. If you're breastfeeding, pump during the day so that you can sleep through at least one feeding. (This strategy doesn't work for everyone. It didn't work for me. Even with a professional turbocharged breast pump, I couldn't get more than an ounce at a time. So, I combined formula feedings earlier than I expected and made a pact with my husband: If I get up for the first 6 months, he has to get up for the next 6 years.)

If you need more motivation to get sleep anywhere and anyhow you can, listen to this: *Sleeping helps you lose weight.* When you're sleep-deprived, fat-storing hormones are released that prevent weight loss. Not only are your fat cells too tired to release fat; you're too tired to move your body and boost your metabolism. But if you make it a priority to get the sleep you need now, you'll be more successful losing weight later. When it comes to weight loss, the saying "you snooze, you lose" has a completely different meaning.

Sleep is something that you need every day, and you need to give to yourself every day. Relatives can fulfill your need for food, your husband can fulfill your need for comfort, your friends can fulfill your need for companionship—*but only you can fulfill your need for sleep.*

Fetal Attraction: Don't Forget to Mother Yourself

When one of my friends jokingly used the term "fetal attraction" to describe a new mother's almost obsessive preoccupation with her baby, I thought it was ingenious. No other term could more accurately describe my baby-on-the-brain existence. After carrying this developing baby for nine months, fantasizing about its look, gender, and personality, as well as fearing for its health and safe delivery into the world—now he was here in the flesh, and I was immediately smitten with maternal love at first sight. If I could bring myself to take my eyes off of that bundle of joy, I was constantly listening for signs of breathing, hunger, and discomfort. If I could bring myself to leave the house without him, I was constantly thinking about him, cutting my errands short, and hurrying home. I got jealous when someone held him for too long (including his father) and anxious when he slept for too long. I joyously announced poopy diapers, giggled when he farted, and uncorked champagne for the shedding of his umbilical cord. I not only didn't care that he spit up in my hair, peed on my clothes, and scratched my face—I thought it was the cutest damn thing that ever happened to me.

No matter how educated, stylish, or cultured I thought I was before having Tyler, I was catapulted back to the primitive level of a mama bear nurturing, protecting, and grooming her baby cub. I no longer cared what I was wearing (nothing fit anyway); as long as he was dressed in a photo-ready outfit, I could be in peace. I no longer cared if I was cleaned, fed, and warm, as long as he was. Makeup disappeared from my bathroom counter, mousse and moisturizer were buried somewhere in the unused drawers, and my jewelry box collected dust. I stopped getting facials, stopped getting my hair cut, and stopped doing my nails.

To tell you the truth, even a year after having Tyler, I had yet to get a facial; I still didn't wear makeup very often, and my nails remained colorless. Part of the deterrent was time—I simply didn't have it. Between writing this book, counseling clients, caring for an active toddler, and maintaining a somewhat sane household, every available minute was occupied. But the other, more important reason was that I no longer had the desire. Motherhood may be hard on the body, but it's easy on the soul. Perspectives change, priorities shift, and life goals transform. Making my body feel good on the inside became more important than making my body look good on the outside, and how I look at the world became infinitely more important than how I look to the world.

So, mothering yourself doesn't necessarily mean styling your hair, polishing your nails, or putting on your face. As with the theme of this chapter, it means taking care of your body from the inside out. You'll have plenty of time to work on the outside later: your figure, hair, skin, nails, and appearance. Right now you need to work on making the inside of your body feel good. You need regular sitz baths, constant rest, sufficient sleep, frequent pad changes, readily available food, clean water, sore muscle relief, and pain management. You also could use someone to cook, clean, open the mail, do the laundry, watch your baby (and your other kids) so you can nap, massage your sore body, kiss away your tears, and comfort your emotions. *Not only do you need to care for yourself, but you also need to feel that other people care about you.*

I remember everyone oohing and aahing over my baby, asking "How's the baby? How old is he? Is he sleeping through the night?" Few people inquired, "How are *you* doing?" When someone did, it brought a big smile to my face—they cared. Now, I make it a point to ask other new mothers how they are doing before I even ask about their babies. And I see the surprised, thankful smile form on their lips.

So, let me ask you: *How are you doing?* Are you recovering from birth? Are you feeling rested? Are you adjusting to your new role as mother? Are you taking care of yourself? Are others caring for you? Are you satisfied with the help you're getting? A study from the University of Minnesota found that the majority of new mothers are satisfied with the outside care and attention they are getting (although in a few weeks you may feel abandoned and dissatisfied, but we'll get to that in the next chapter). So, take advantage of it now and let others mother you. Welcome your mother-in-law with open arms (as long as she can cook), ask your mother to stay an extra week, accept offers of food and help from friends and neighbors, or hire some help if you don't have family and friends nearby. Or, if you're getting too much outside help and need more peace, quiet, and bonding time, say so. Ask your mother-in-law to stay in a hotel (or better yet, have your husband ask her), and request that your mother come back for a longer stay in a month or so. Just make sure your needs are met—whether they're for support or solitude.

Most important, apply some of your own mothering instinct to yourself. As women and mothers, we are innate healers, emotionally attuned to our surroundings, and blessed with a healing touch. In some countries, men even wear feminine attire to try to summon their mothering instinct and healing powers. Of course, no matter what they wear, they'll always come up short in the mothering department because they weren't born with the nurturing gene. This recently identified gene increases our sight, sound, and smell acuities for infants, as well as enhances our fine motor skills so that we can care for these fragile, miniature beings. How many men have you heard say that they love the smell of babies? How many men have you seen sit upright in bed at the sound of a barely audible gurgle? How many men have you witnessed expertly cutting those tiny fingernails or changing a newborn diaper? Once we tell them that the baby is up, they may be able to easily find their way to the crib because of their keen sense of direction, but once they get there, they stare at the diaper for a while, not knowing which end is up.

As the Jewish proverb states, "God couldn't be everywhere so he (she?) created mothers." It's an honor to be God's right-hand woman with our amazing mothering instinct—we just have to remember to mother ourselves. And we can begin the process of mothering ourselves with these four simple words: *What do I need?* Ninety percent of the time the answer will probably be sleep, but you may very well discover that what you need is:

- a healthy, nutritious meal
- a glass of cool, refreshing water
- a massage for your sore muscles
- some pain medication for your afterbirth contractions
- a long, relaxing sitz bath
- some quality time with a good friend
- to stay home in your pajamas all day and nest with your baby
- to get out of the house and reacquaint yourself with the world
- to accept help and offers of food from family and friends
- to ask for help from family and friends

"I know what I need!" exclaimed Tammy. "No more visitors! People are constantly stopping by to see the baby, and I'm entertaining them more than I'm caring for myself." I know the feeling. I remember getting phone calls from people saying they were on their way and would be stopping by in fifteen minutes. I would rush from room to room picking up, throw on some clothes, put on some makeup, and put on a fake smile as I opened the door. Then I got wise. Even if I was showered and dressed, I'd mess up my hair, put on a bathrobe, and yawn every two minutes to cut their visit short. Then I got even wiser and started telling them, "This isn't a good time to visit; I was about to take a nap."

As Vicki Iovine recommends in *The Girlfriend's Guide to Surviving the First Year of Motherhood* (a great book that every new mother should read), "Don't stand when you can sit, don't sit when you can lie down, and don't stay awake when you can sleep." Perhaps the best advice I've heard for the first few weeks. I'd like to add: eat well, drink plenty of water, enjoy your baby, and get together with people you love—even if it means letting the house get dirty, letting your hair dry itself, letting the mail pile up, and letting the birth announcements wait. Your baby certainly won't care, and neither will most people. They'll understand—you just had a baby and deserve to do anything (or not do anything) you damn well please.

The work, chores, and obligations will always be there, but your newborn won't. With what seems like a blink of an eye they go from infancy to adolescence, from diapers to dating, and from carriage to college. Ask any mother of older children what they remember of those first few weeks and what they would do differently if they could relive it. I haven't come across one who wishes she had eaten less, exercised more, kept the house cleaner, or sent out the birth announcements sooner. The only wish I've heard is to go back to that magical time with a more relaxed attitude and fewer obligations, and to enjoy every single minute with her beautiful new baby.

What's Your Postpartum Peace Plan for the First Six Weeks?

This chapter had little to do with losing pregnancy fat because your fat cells will have nothing to do with shrinking in the first six weeks. Instead, the focus was on you—your recovery, your needs, and your health. Now it's time for you to choose what you'll focus on to nurture yourself as you're nurturing your baby. In other words, what's your postpartum peace plan for these first six weeks? What will you do to pamper, eat, actively move, calm your life, and embrace your body? Check all that you feel will enhance your postpartum recovery.

What Will You Do to Pamper Yourself?

____ I will enjoy the magical first six weeks.

____ I will relieve pain with ice packs, sitz baths, massage and/or medication if I need it.

____ I will nap when my baby naps.

____ I will accept offerings of food and help.
____ I will let others mother me.
____ I will apply some of my own mothering instinct to myself.
____ I will repeatedly ask: What do I need?

What Will You Do to Eat With a Regular Meal Schedule?

____ I won't even think about dieting.
____ I will eat basically the same way I did when I was pregnant.
____ I will keep taking my prenatal supplements.
____ I will drink water throughout the day.

What Will You Do to Actively Move Your Body?

____ I will exercise my right not to exercise.
____ I will do my tummy sucks and Kegel exercises.
____ I will take short walks with my baby.
____ I will check my diastasis to see when it's safe to start doing crunches.
____ I will define exercise loosely—anytime I'm moving, I'm exercising, and that includes changing diapers, opening gifts, and going out to get the mail.

What Will You Do to Calm Your Stress?

____ I will realize that the baby blues is real, normal, and will heal just like the rest of my body.
____ I will seek help if my depression lasts more than two weeks.
____ I will turn off the phone ringer and disconnect the doorbell to maintain my peace and privacy.
____ I will decline visitors when I don't want them.
____ I will invite family and friends over when I need to socialize.

What Will You Do to Embrace Your New Body?

____ I will acknowledge my body's strength and power.

____ I will be grateful that my body is programmed to heal from the inside out.

____ I will realize that my body has already lost significant weight on its own, and fat loss will soon follow.

Chapter Five

The Next Six Weeks: Getting Back on Your Feet

Well, the first six weeks flew by with a blink of an eye, and I'm proud to announce that I not only made it through my initiation into motherhood, but that I'm also an expert diaper changer, burper, bather, and breastfeeder. I'm still feeling a bit sore and very tired, but my doctor says that everything looks A-OK below the belt and that I can 'resume normal sexual, social, and physical activity' again. My husband was thrilled with the news, but I wanted to go barricade myself in a closet and never come out. My friends say not to worry, all new mothers are tentative the first time they have sex, go out to a party without their babies, or venture out to a gym to burn away the pregnancy fat. They tell me that life will 'go back to normal' in no time. Is that true?"

First of all, there is no "going back." You are a different person today than you were a few months ago. You have a baby, you are a mother, and your life will be forever changed with unprecedented joy and unexpected difficulties. Second, there is no such thing as "normal." What was normal in your prebaby days—a normal schedule, a normal exercise program, a normal night's sleep, a normal social life, and a normal sex life—seem almost laughable now. Your routine changes more often than the weather, your baby has no predictable eating or sleeping schedule (and therefore neither do you), and your nighttime activities are still limited to breastfeeding, reading your newborn books, and passing on your husband's advances in order to pass out on the couch. But despite the absence of normalcy, most of my clients can't imagine going back to a life sans baby. They would much rather wake up to their baby's cries than to the buzzing alarm clock, and they would much prefer taking care of their babies than taking care of business. Even if time travel were possible, they wouldn't turn back the clock to their childless days. Would you? What was considered "normal" back then seems very abnormal today, because you wouldn't have your baby in your life.

Your life is different now, with a different definition of normal, and like your life, your body probably feels forever altered, too. Even though your doctor may have told you that you're fully recovered, your body is telling you otherwise. And I'm not just talking about your weight, shape, and size. I'm referring to your energy, strength, balance, vaginal tissue, and sexual desire. Researchers at the University of Washington School of Nursing found that at six weeks postpartum, 80 percent of us still used words like "sore," "tired," and "exhausted" to describe our physical state. Even at the end of a year, vaginal discomfort, decreased sex drive, hemorrhoids, night sweats, and fatigue still persist in some of us.

How would you describe your physical state right now? Do you feel fully recovered? Do you have the energy and stamina to work up a sweat in either the bedroom or the workout room? I know I didn't at six weeks. My joints ached, I was still spotting some blood, I was flat-out exhausted, and I was cringing at the thought of sex. Even though I was deemed recovered as far as my medical records were concerned, my body was still in the midst of repair and stayed there for weeks to come. A small handful of you may feel physically fantastic and ready to take on the world, but the remaining four out of five will feel just like I did—not quite up to par and not quite ready to partake in physically demanding and psychologically taxing activities (including but not limited to exercise, intercourse, house cleaning, meal preparation, clothes shopping, hair maintenance, and primping for social events).

Although this chapter is about helping you to get back on your feet, increase your activity level, and start a structured, purposeful exercise program to burn away the pregnancy fat, you may not feel ready. And that's perfectly acceptable, at least for right now. In fact, if your body is signaling rest instead of movement, I encourage you to stay off your feet for a few more weeks—it won't make a bit of difference to your long-term success in postbaby weight loss. There are no hard-and-fast rules when it comes to outsmarting your postpartum fat cells, just soft, slow recommendations.

On Your Mark, Get Set . . . Stop

Remember Jackie from the last chapter? She was the overanxious exerciser who couldn't wait to start. As soon as she got the thumbs-up to exercise from her OB at her six-week checkup, she drove straight to the gym for a two-hour, heart-pounding workout, then vowed to go every day until she lost every ounce of weight. By the sixth day of running, biking, rowing, stair climbing, and weight lifting, her vaginal bleeding started again, her weakness and pain came back, and her baby started to turn the other cheek to her breast milk. Because she jumped off the exercise starting block doing too much too soon, she set back her body's recovery and had to wait another month before she could start an exercise program again—one that was easier on her body and kinder to her baby this time around.

For those of you who are also poised to go full speed ahead with exercise, I urge you to picture a stop sign, then proceed with caution. Start slowly and stop if your body (or your baby) tells you that you are doing too much. For example:

- If your bleeding starts again or if it turns from brown to bright red . . . *stop!* It's a red flag (so to speak) that the physical stress and movement are causing trauma to your still healing uterus.

- If you feel light-headed or dizzy . . . *stop!* Your body fluids are still adjusting and too much of your blood supply is being directed to your muscles and away from your brain.

- If you feel pain in your joints or muscles . . . *stop!* Your center of gravity is still out of balance and your muscles and joints haven't realigned themselves yet.

- If your baby doesn't want to nurse after you exercise . . . *stop!* Even though the breastfeeding–exercise research has shown inconsistent results, it appears that some babies don't like the taste of breastmilk after a long, hard workout. Lactic acid is released during strenuous exercise, and although it hasn't been found to harm babies in any way, it can leave a bad taste in their mouth, and they may refuse to nurse. Exercise is good for you; breastfeeding is good for the baby—but the combination may not be great for either of you. You do have options: You can slow down the pace of your workouts, time your workouts for after you've breastfed, and/or cut your workouts short (your baby may not like you to be away for so long, anyway).

- If you're about to start some heavy weight training . . . *stop!* Give yourself another few weeks before you lift weights. Your muscles and joints aren't quite ready for it yet.

- If you're doing a hundred or more sit-ups a day . . . *stop!* Check your diastasis, as described in chapter 4, to make sure it's closed because in about 10 percent of you, it isn't yet. Even if your abdominal muscles have healed back together, one hundred crunches are too many. An exercise physiologist once shared with me a good rule of thumb: Only do as many sit-ups as you are days postpartum. Which means you shouldn't be even close to one hundred until the next chapter, where I'll discuss ab work in more detail.

- If you plan to go back to your prepregnancy workout schedule . . . *stop!* You're not ready to rejoin your kickboxing class, tennis club, or power-walking group that meets four days a week. You may be ready to meet your walking pals one or two days a week, but you probably wouldn't be able to keep up with them anyway.

- If you haven't gotten the okay from your OB . . . *stop!* Don't assume you can automatically start exercising when you reach six weeks, and if you had a C-section or a very difficult labor, don't be surprised if your doctor tells you to hold off for a few more weeks. Listen to his or her wisdom, your doctor really does know best.

Easing into exercise is vital for your health and recovery. But you may not need these words of caution if starting is more of a problem than stopping. And starting was a huge obstacle for another of my clients, Susie. Unlike my exercise enthusiast, Jackie, she was an exercise avoidist. She had never once joined an aerobics class, never did a leg lift or sit-up in her life, never walked anywhere unless it was absolutely necessary (like the time she ran out of gas on the highway and had to hoof it to the nearest gas station), and never bought a pair of sneakers, athletic socks, or a sports bra, which was her way of boycotting the fitness movement. Needless to say, Susie was not looking forward to starting a postpartum exercise program, and was my toughest antiexercise client ever. Whenever I brought up the e-word, she would retort with comments like, "I'd rather have a root canal! I'd rather save my pennies for liposuction! I'd rather wait for a miracle fat-burning pill!"

You may not be as adamantly antiexercise as Susie, but there's a very good chance that you, too, are less than thrilled about starting a postpartum exercise program. Before having a baby 60 percent of you didn't exercise at all, and another 20 percent didn't exercise consistently enough to make a difference—so I wouldn't be surprised if you have some resistance. Few new mothers hold the attitude that they "can't wait to exercise." Most can wait, and unfortunately most wait too long. You can wait a few weeks, but not months and years. If you don't start moving your body soon and keep it moving regularly over the next nine months, you may find yourself struggling with postpregnancy pounds when your baby is getting her postdoctorate degree. *This is your opportunity to start to get your body back in shape, and you can't do it without exercise.* You may think that your body will miraculously lose weight on its own, but it won't. You may pray that one day you'll simply wake up, walk into your closet, and fit into all of your prepregnancy clothes, but that day will never dawn. Unless, of course, you exercise. If you want to lose those pesky, persnickety, postpartum pounds, you have to come to your body's aid, make peace with your fat cells, and make exercise a part of your life. You have no other choice.

If there was any other way to outsmart your postpartum fat cells, I'd be the first to share it with you. My life's work has been dedicated to female fat cells, and over twenty years' experience with thousands of women has made me a devout believer in the fat-burning power of exercise. Still, there are women out there who doubt the necessity of exercise, disbelievers who are in a futile search for make believe exercise. And there are plenty of companies out there who fuel their search with pills and gadgets that promise "weight loss without exercise." A recent alluring easy-way-out of exercise is electrical muscle stimulation. It sounds great; you lie down on a bed, close your eyes, and let the electrical impulses fool your muscles into thinking that they're running a marathon. But as with anything in life, if it sounds too good to be true, it probably is. Your muscles are no fools, they know the difference between electrical shock and walking around the block. They can detect whether you're really exercising or just pretending to be.

Sometime during these next six weeks, *all* of you, including Susie, will be physically ready to start a real exercise program. My mission is to also get you psychologically ready—to get your head in the right place so that you will successfully get your body in shape. And, you'll be happy to hear, this psychological preparation doesn't involve moving a muscle. No walking, no leg lifts, no stair climbing, no sit-ups, no working out—only head work. If you take the time to think about what you'll do, when you'll do it, and how you'll keep doing it, you'll be infinitely more successful than the average woman who calls it quits after just three weeks of an exercise program. That average woman didn't have a realistic plan before she started. She didn't choose an activity that she enjoyed (or at least tolerated), and she didn't set an exercise schedule that she could stick with.

If you are a past example of this average woman, repeatedly starting an exercise program only to throw in the towel before you've had a chance to use it to wipe off the sweat, I want to make you well above average this time. I want you to be exercising thirty years from now, never mind three weeks from now. That's why I want you to spend some time pondering these three questions:

1. What will you do?
2. When will you do it?
3. Why will you keep doing it?

They are your psychological tools for exercise success, and therefore, weight loss success.

What Will You Do?

Most of my clients' first response to this question is to "join a club"—a reasonable answer for anyone in search of a fit body. But unless the health club is a block away and offers child care, it's unreasonable to assume you'll have the two-hour block of time it takes to get there, work out, shower, and get back to your hungry baby who is desperate for a breast. You'll be lucky if you make it more than a couple of times before deciding that the hefty membership fee was a waste of money. There are twenty-two million of us who belong to a health club, and twenty-six million of us who used to belong to one. You may very well be one of these twenty-six million ex–health club members, and if you couldn't get yourself there before having a child, the chances of making it past the registration desk now are even slimmer. Unless you know beyond a shadow of a doubt that you're the type of person who needs to go to a fitness-oriented establishment to work out or you won't do it, other options may be more realistic right now.

Like investing in a piece of home exercise equipment? Once my clients realize that the odds are against them making it to the gym, they think the next best thing is to bring the gym to them by buying a treadmill, stair climber, rowing machine, stationary bike, or other newfangled workout apparatus. But according to the Fitness Products Council, 35 percent of us only use home exercise equipment a few times before it becomes a clothes hanger, and 8 percent of us barely take it out of the box, never using it even once before it's abandoned in the garage. Whether the unused exercise equipment is covered with clothes or cobwebs, it becomes a constant reminder that we failed at fitness.

We are *not* fitness failures. *We didn't fail in our attempts at starting an exercise program; the exercise program failed us*. I've owned exercise equipment, only to sell it or give it away because it was taking up valuable space. I belong to a health club, and I'm lucky if I make it there once a week (as I write this, I think it's been more than two weeks since I've shown my face in the workout room). And I know I'm not an exercise failure. I've been exercising for twenty-four years of my life—I'm an exercise success story because I've changed my program to my ever-changing lifestyle. I began decades ago with running when my youthful knees and college schedule were conducive to pounding the pavement, then I switched to racquetball when my competitive nature needed an outlet, then I became an aerobic dance groupie when it was hip to hang out with my single friends at the club, then I joined a low-key neighborhood gym where I could work out in baggy sweats and complete solitude. And since I've had Tyler, I've changed my exercise program once again—I walk three or four days a week with him on the hiking trails in the Oakland hills. This new program suits my new lifestyle and my new needs, which are to be with my baby, to get out of the house, and to be stimulated by the fresh air and beauty of Mother Nature.

My guess is that your needs are similar. A new mother and her baby are joined at the hip (as well as the breast) and need inseparable physical closeness. A new mother and her baby need to get out of the house where they have been nesting for the last six weeks. And a new mother and her baby need sunlight, fresh air, and movement. If babies could be surveyed, they would no doubt rate outdoor walks as their favorite activity; the fresh air first perks them up, then the movement lulls them to sleep. I remember when I first started walking with my peanut-sized Tyler in a front baby carrier. For the first half of the walk, he would be cooing with delight and I would be smiling from ear to ear as I listened to his adorable sounds. For the second half, he would be in a deep, restful sleep on my chest, and I would be immersed in my own deep thoughts. Both of us were, and still are, in walking heaven. Unfortunately, he no longer fits comfortably in a front baby carrier (which we both miss), but the backpack or jogger keeps both of us dedicated to our walking schedules.

At least for this first year, walking with your baby is the winning ticket for weight loss. Research has found that women who walk with their babies lose more weight, more quickly than women who try to exercise when their babies are asleep or when they have child care. One of the reasons is that both moms and babies find walking enjoyable, so they are more likely to do it. Another, equally important reason is that there is less of a chance something is going to get in the way of your walk. The weather may put a damper on your outdoor excursion, but you can always go to the mall and do a lap or two before you run your errands. If, instead, you try to exercise when you have child care or when your baby is napping, more than the weather is bound to interfere. The refrigerator was empty, and you had to go to the grocery store, the line at the post office took up your exercise time, your fourth grader needed a present for his friend's birthday party, the car needed an oil change, the dry cleaning needed to be dropped off, the bills needed to be paid, the taxes needed to get done, the house needed to be cleaned, the phone calls needed to be returned—the list of potential exercise interferers is endless, which means you're significantly less likely to do it.

Although I am obviously a strong advocate of walking with your baby, *the bottom line is that you just have to get off your bottom and move*. Take a yoga class, sweep your deck, do a postpartum exercise video, dance around the house with your baby, wrestle on the floor with your older kids, pace while you're talking on the phone, walk up and down the stairs, and fidget whenever possible. The Mayo clinic recently published a phenomenal finding: People who fidget can burn up to an extra seven hundred calories a day just by not sitting still. That's the equivalent of walking about eight miles a day!

Walking isn't limited to the outdoors anymore. The latest fitness craze is simply walking around your house—your kitchen, bedroom, bathroom, laundry room, and diaper-changing table—counting the number of steps you take each day. There are even nifty little pedometers that you can strap on to your body and let the steps click away. The goal for health and weight loss is taking between eight thousand to ten thousand steps a day. If that sounds like a lot of walking to you, it's because it is. The average sedentary American takes only about two thousand steps a day; most of our time is spent sitting in the car, sitting at our desk, and sitting in front of the computer and television. And since you've given birth, you've been sitting a lot more than you've been stepping. You've been sitting to breastfeed, sitting to bottle-feed, sitting to rock, sitting to cuddle, and sitting to rest because you're not getting enough sleep. *If you keep sitting around, you'll stay round.* So, get up and move: Get up to answer the phone instead of keeping the portable handset by your side, get up to check on your baby instead of having a monitor in every room, and get up to go shopping instead of having the Internet run your errands for you.

You may have to consciously get up and move your body today, but as the months fly by and your baby becomes an active toddler, you won't have to consciously do anything. Your lifestyle will automatically become more conducive to stepping away the pounds. I've never seen a study on the number of steps a mother of a toddler takes in a day, but I wore a pedometer one day trying to keep up with my off-and-running Tyler who never sits still, and I chalked up almost twelve thousand steps without even leaving the house.

But you can't wait until your baby is a toddler to outsmart your postpartum fat cells. *You have to take your first step before your baby does.* As a Chinese proverb states, "A journey of a thousand miles begins with a single step." You may feel a thousand pounds away from your weight goals, but all you have to do is take your first step. In fact, you've already taken your first step by reading this chapter and thinking about what you'll do to get fit. If you want to take your second step, put down this book and walk around the house, go up and down the stairs, take a stroll around the block, or put on some music and dance. There's no better time than right now.

When Will You Do It?

If your goal is to wake up an hour earlier to exercise before your baby wakes up, good luck. Your need for sleep is greater than your need for movement, and the warm comfortable bed and snooze button within arm's reach will almost always win over exercise. If you plan to do it when your husband or partner gets home from work, good luck. By the end of the day, you're exhausted, and your need for adult time may be greater than your need for exercise. Therefore, your best bet is to do it sometime during the day—anytime during the day—anytime you can spare a few minutes. If you only have five or ten minutes to move, you can get down on the floor and do some leg-lifts or get out the vacuum and push with a vengeance. If you have the luxury of twenty or more minutes, you can go out for a walk with your baby in tow or pop the postpartum exercise video into the VCR.

Every purposeful movement makes a difference and every minute adds up. That's right. The latest exercise research has given us new mothers something to cheer about. As you start your fitness program, you don't have to exercise continuously for thirty-plus minutes to see some initial change in your body. You just have to move your body throughout the day so that the total time adds up to a half hour or more—and you'll be doing enough to start gaining strength and losing weight. Do I hear you cheering? Not if you've been banking on the "I don't have time to exercise" excuse. With this new research from the Cooper Institute in Dallas and other facilities throughout the nation, every new mother now has the time to embark on an exercise program. All it takes is five minutes here, ten minutes there, and a walk with your baby a few days a week. Later on down the road, you'll need to exercise longer and continuously to burn away the pregnancy fat, but we'll cross that bridge when we come to it. Right now, just focus on getting on the road and staying there for as many minutes as you can.

Why Will You Keep Doing It?

The obvious answer may be to lose the pregnancy weight, but as you now know, your exercise program won't lead to significant weight loss for another month or two. Your fat cells are just waking up from their postbirth hibernation, and it will take them a while to become fully functional. But there is a reason to start exercising sooner rather than later. Exercising now may not force them to shrink, but it will jolt them awake so they can start to manufacture the fat-releasing enzymes. None of these enzymes were formed in the first six weeks, some can be manufactured now, but the majority will be made and activated after the three-month point.

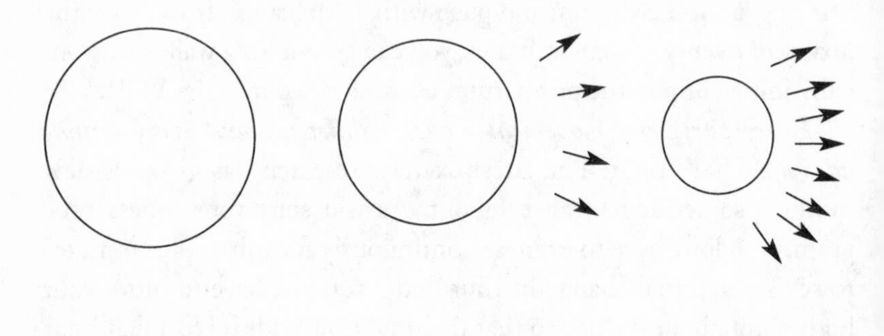

First Six Weeks Second Six Weeks Next Six Months

Then, why should you even lift a finger until after three months? Because you'll still be increasing your future fat-burning potential, setting yourself up to be more efficient and successful at shrinking your fat cells later. In the long term, weight loss will keep you motivated—those who exercise lose a third more weight over a year—but in the short term, it's important to find other immediate rewards that are important to you. So why will you keep exercising?

- **For more energy?** Exercise increases your blood circulation and breathing rate, which brings more nutrients and oxygen to your brain and all your other organs and cells. Even ten minutes of exercise has been found to increase energy levels by 25 percent. Think about it: A little movement gives you significantly more energy to care for your baby and yourself.

- **For a better mood?** Exercise stimulates the release of endorphins and serotonin in our brains, which stabilize our moods. And the rhythmic motion of exercise is a form of meditation, which reduces our stress. In addition, the University of Michigan found that postpartum women who exercise report having more fun in their lives—more socializing, more entertaining, and more shopping. Don't girls just want to have fun? Especially more fun while shopping?

- **For a better sex life?** The University of Texas found that as little as twenty minutes of exercise increased sexual responsiveness in women (much more so than in men), presumably due to increased blood flow. Who would have thought exercise could be an aphrodisiac, helping you to overcome the sex jitters? Mention this bit of research to your husband, and you may find that a personal trainer has moved into your house.

- **For a better world?** Women who start exercising to support a cause they believe in are likely to keep doing it. Training for a walk, run, or bike ride for breast cancer, AIDS, battered women, the homeless, or other important cause gives you a feeling of accomplishment and the motivation to keep moving.

- **For a longer life?** The University of Minnesota School of Public Health followed forty thousand women and found that those who exercised just once a week were 24 percent less likely to die prematurely than those who didn't exercise at all. Don't we all want to prevent an early death? We want to be a part of our children's and grandchildren's lives for as long as we can.

Speaking of children, they may be the most powerful exercise motivator of all. So powerful that it was the only trigger that ejected my toughest antiexercise client ever, Susie, off her duff. She wasn't the least bit moved by aspirations to a better world, better sex, or a better mood. But as soon as I shared some research proving that when a mother makes exercise a part of her life, her children are 50 percent more likely to value fitness and be physically active, she went out and bought her first pair of sneakers. It took her over a month to actually put them on, but she finally did it to be an active role model for her daughter. And eight years later, she's still walking—and her daughter is playing soccer, swimming, and riding her bike whenever she can.

What's your powerful motivator? Find it and pick a start date over the next few weeks. It doesn't matter if you start a week from now or a month from now. All that matters is that you start.

STILL EATING FOR TWO?

After telling you to eat the same way as you did in pregnancy for the past six weeks, it's time to switch gears and help you eat like you did before you got pregnant (or if you've been overeating for most of your life, to help you eat like you've never eaten before). Up until now, you needed the extra calories and nutrients for tissue repair, recovery, and for your breast milk to come in. But from now on, your body no longer needs the huge meals, hot fudge sundaes, and all-you-can-eat buffets. And when your body doesn't need something, it goes straight to your fat cells for storage.

It's true. While you're trying to lose weight in the postpartum months, your eating can actually make you gain weight. One study found that after an initial postbirth weight loss of seventeen to twenty pounds, some women can reverse direction and gain three or four pounds in these next six weeks. The reason: They were overeating and storing the excess calories in their fat cells. And it's not just hot fudge sundaes that get stored in your fat cells faster than the speed of light. Fat is the storage form of every food: bread and bananas, fish and fowl, cantaloupe and carrots, tofu and tomatoes. In other words, you can gain weight regardless of how healthily you're eating. *You can gain weight from eating healthy foods in unhealthy portions.*

Do I have your attention? No woman wants to gain weight after having a baby, but that could be your fate if you're still eating for two. Not to worry. This section will prevent any and all additional weight gain and will ensure a weight-loss future, because I'm going to help you go *from eating for two to eating for you.*

It's not as easy as you may think. After eating larger meals, frequent snacks, and nighttime treats for the past forty or fifty weeks, overeating has become a habit. You may be grabbing food, eating sweets, and taking second helpings without a second thought. And habits take time and effort to break. Research has found that it takes at least six weeks for new habits to replace old ones—that's why these next six weeks are the perfect time frame to break your overeating habits and replace them with more moderate ones.

So, think about the eating habits you formed during pregnancy. Some may be quite positive, like eating more fresh foods, organic produce, and dairy products. These are obviously habits you want to keep. Others, however, are not worth keeping because they work against your weight loss efforts. I polled about three hundred new mothers on the pregnancy eating habits that became their problematic postpartum eating habits. Here are the four most common answers:

- **"I developed a sweet tooth."** Most pregnant women gravitate toward sugar; I know I did. When you were pregnant, your body knew that high-sugar foods provided the concentrated calories to help your baby grow. But now the calorie-packed cookies, cakes, pastries, and sweets will only help your fat cells grow.

- **"I snack every night before bed."** When you were pregnant, your body's exploding metabolism stimulated your appetite morning, noon, and night; and your after-hours appetite was a welcomed opportunity to indulge in a guilt-free midnight treat. But now your metabolism has hit rock bottom, so what you eat late at night is no longer "for the baby"; it's for your fat cells. And they are quite pleased with your continued nighttime nibbling.

- **"I have a huge dinner every night followed by a good-sized dessert."** Dinner has always been our biggest meal of the day, and during pregnancy, that nighttime meal reached record proportions. Big dinners lead to bigger fat cells. And if they are followed by big desserts, they lead to even bigger, and happier, fat cells.

- **"I eat a supersized chocolate bar every afternoon."** The number one craved food during pregnancy is chocolate; the number one craved food during the postpartum period is chocolate; the number one craved food by women of any age during any chosen moment is chocolate. So, postpartum or not, it's no wonder this habit is etched in stone. But do you need a huge bar? Wouldn't a small piece do the trick? And do you really need it every day? When I asked these questions to Catherine (also known as the Queen of Chocolate to her friends), she replied, "I probably don't need a jumbo bar every day, so I've decided to get a handle on my chocolate cravings. I'm only going to let myself eat a regular size bar on days that end in the letter *y*." Progress, but she still had some work to do, so I recommended that Cathy read *Outsmarting Female Food Cravings,* a book I wrote to help women effectively manage their chocolate cravings. After spending some time digesting the information, she called me up and said, "Okay, I get it now. I'm only going to eat a third of a small size chocolate bar on days that don't begin with the letter *b*."

Other, troublesome habits that started in pregnancy and stuck in the postpartum months included eating while driving in the car, waking up in the middle of the night to graze in the kitchen, and eating off of other people's plates. Yes, some women became plate-pickers, and their rationale was that the calories rightfully belonged to the owner of the plate, and therefore, clung to the china, preventing the transfer of the calories to their own bodies.

What pregnancy eating habits do you think are interfering with your postpartum weight-loss efforts? What rationale do you have for keeping them? That you need the energy boost from the sugar because you're so tired? Sugar may give you a twenty- or thirty-minute temporary boost, but then your energy plummets to an all-time low. That you need the hundreds of extra calories from big dinners and desserts because you're breastfeeding full time? According to some recent research from the Netherlands and elsewhere, the caloric cost of breastfeeding may be lower than previously thought, which means that the recommended five hundred extra calories for breastfeeding mothers may be too high. If you're breastfeeding, please don't interpret this research to mean that you can restrict calories and skip meals. You can't. You still need to eat, and you still need to eat regularly. The question is: *How much do you need to eat?* Do you need the heaping plate of pasta or would a smaller serving satisfy your body's needs? Do you need the entire bag of potato chips or would a handful do the trick? Do you need a chocolate fudge sundae or would a scoop of ice cream put a smile on your face?

What most postpartum women need is a crash course on putting their portions in proportion. Do you know the definition of a standard portion size? It's the amount of food your body needs to function for the next few hours and it's smaller than you ever imagined—usually a small fraction of what's found in the bag or box, what you serve yourself, or what is served to you. For example, a restaurant serving of pasta, a Cracker Jack box, a submarine sandwich, and a twelve-inch pizza each contain about four standard, individual-sized portions. But we eat them thinking they are single servings made just for us, when in fact they could theoretically feed a family of four.

No wonder obesity in America is reaching epidemic levels; our out-of-control portions have led to out-of-control weight gain. And during pregnancy, there was no limit to the amount some of us packed into our bodies—a one-pound bag of chips for a snack, two sandwiches at lunch, a sixteen-inch pizza for dinner. *To reduce the size of our bodies, we have to reduce the size of our portions.* Here are a few other standard portion sizes to help you realize just how much you've been overeating.

4 to 8 crackers (depending on size)
½ of an English muffin
½ cup of fruit juice
¼ cup of cottage cheese
1 egg
10 peanuts
1 slice of bacon
⅛ of an avocado

When was the last time you had one egg and one measly slice of bacon? Or stopped at ten tiny peanuts? Or put an eighth of an avocado, a couple of small slivers, on your salad or sandwich? Or walked away after just four crackers? If they were of the nonfat variety, you probably stayed put and ate the entire box. Just check out the nutrition labels of packaged foods, and you'll see how many single servings are in that single box or bag—it's definitely not one, and may be a dozen or more.

I realize that, at first glance, these portion sizes seem ridiculously small, and I don't necessarily expect you to survive on one-quarter cup of cottage cheese or one-half cup of fruit juice. But I do expect you to make the connection between extra-large portion sizes and extra-large fat cells. It's simple mathematics: If you eat a ton of food, you'll gain a ton of weight. This mathematical theory was tested and proven by you during your pregnancy. Don't bother testing it during the postpartum period. It's already been established: If you keep eating a ton of food, you'll not only hold on to a ton of weight, you'll keep gaining more weight.

We can blame our weight struggles, pregnancy related or not, on our portion distortion. And we can blame our portion distortion on restaurants, fast food establishments, and the snack industry. Many of the portion sizes have increased more than 200 percent in the past twenty years. Take a bagel for example. It used to be a two-ounce mini-bagel; now it's a five to seven ounce monstrosity containing four hundred to six hundred calories (and that's before the cream cheese!). A standard portion of steak is three ounces, and a big steak used to be ten or twelve ounces; but now some restaurants boast sixteen- , twenty-two- , or even thirty-six-ounce slabs of beef. With that much cow, muumuus are bound to come back in style. And what ever happened to twelve-ounce sodas? Now they are poured into a twenty- or even thirty-two-ounce cup. Big Gulps, supersized meals, industrial-sized packages of snack foods from warehouse stores—*supersized foods have run amok and taken our weights with them.*

To end your weight struggles, you have to end your portion distortion. If you automatically eat what's in the bag, in the box, or on your plate, your big portions will keep you a big postpartum woman. But if you think before you eat and visually estimate a regular portion size, you'll become a regular-sized woman again. The following chart should help you eyeball a portion size first, and eat second.

Use your eyes to estimate a small portion of a particular food and use your hand to get a handle on the definition of a small meal. A handful of food is almost always enough to fuel your body without filling your fat cells. Think of your last meal or snack: Could you have fit it into your hand? Or would it have filled two or three handfuls? Most women find that they are eating two or three times the amount their bodies need—that triple decker club sandwich, overflowing plate of pasta primavera, or package of SnackWells cookies couldn't possibly fit into one hand. If it can't fit into your hand, it can't fit into your stomach without signaling to your brain that you're overeating and stimulating your fat cells to store the extra calories as fat.

A Regular Portion Is	And the Size of
1 medium-sized fruit	A tennis ball
½ cup of fruit or vegetable	An ice-cream scoop
1 medium-sized baked potato	A computer mouse
¾ cup of cereal	A handful
½ cup of pasta, rice, corn, or polenta	A fist
2-ounce bagel	A yo-yo
1 tablespoon of butter, margarine, peanut butter, or mayonnaise	A thumb tip
1 ounce of cheese	A checker
3 ounces of meat	A deck of cards
1 pancake	A CD
1 slice of bread	A CD jacket
1 slice of deli meat	A floppy disk

By this time, most of my clients get the "smaller portion, smaller meal" hint, but they have a pressing question: *What foods am I supposed to be eating in those smaller portions and meals?* And they are perturbed with my rather vague answer, which is "anything you want." Vague or not, it's true. You can eat anything you want in small portions, and it won't sabotage your weight loss efforts because you're never overeating and never stimulating your fat cells to store. *What you eat doesn't matter; how much you eat does.* Carbohydrates don't make you fat; eating loaves of bread, pounds of pasta, and bushels of potatoes does. Fat doesn't make you fat; eating bottles of salad dressing, jars of mayonnaise, and sticks of butter does.

But I'm getting ahead of myself. I'll discuss more of the what-to-eat information in the next chapter, so for right now, let go of any eating angst and just keep eating the same things you have been eating in smaller portions. You need to eat to lose weight, and you need to eat to provide the energy to start exercising, start resuming your social life, and start having sex again. But it may take a good deal more than food and energy to jump-start your sex life.

Who Put the Hex on Sex?

"If my husband tries to have sex with me one more time, I may have to go in search of one of those old chastity belts. I'm scared it will hurt, I don't feel at all sexual, our baby is still sleeping in the room with us, and three definitely is a crowd."

Sound familiar? You may not have contemplated chastity belts, but the idea doesn't sound too bad. Your sexual activity probably decreased throughout your pregnancy, may have been nonexistent during the last trimester, and has been forbidden for the last six weeks. It's almost like having sex for the very first time again. Only this time, you don't have butterflies of excitement in your stomach, you have knots in your stomach, stitches in the tissue surrounding your vagina, and hemorrhoids in the area around your anus. No wonder your interest in sex has reached an all-time low.

Who put the hex on sex? Probably Mother Nature. She intended to make you a cold fish for a while with decreased sex drive, sore tissue, and lack of lubrication. Her goal is to make sure you don't get pregnant again too quickly, knowing that it would be too taxing on your body and your sanity. Could you imagine getting pregnant right now? Occasionally it happens; ovulation can occur before we start our periods. That's why your OB talked about birth control at your six-week checkup, but Mother Nature doesn't know about the medical advancements of birth control pills, diaphragms, IUDs, and vasectomies. She only knows her own method of birth control—decreased sex drive.

Mother Nature will lift her antisex curse and your sex drive will return, maybe even to a heightened level of intensity, but it may take a while. Even at six months, 50 percent of us report having less interest in sex. By that time our bodies should be ready and raring to go for marathon sex, so maybe it's our minds that aren't ready. What is your mind telling you about after-the-baby sex?

- That you're a mother, and mothers don't have wild, passionate sex?
- That sex wasn't great before you had a baby, and now you're afraid that the fireworks will be gone forever?
- That your husband hates your body, and doesn't find you attractive any more?
- That you hate your body, and you would die if your husband saw your naked body with the lights on?

You won't die, but your husband's probably dying to see your naked body, and would die and go to heaven if you initiated sex and abandoned yourself in the act with complete body acceptance. Just ask him. Most men report that they actually prefer the full curves and ample breasts of the postpartum women in their lives—and although sex is high on their wish list, they understand their partners' postbaby tentativeness. Some even have a sense of humor about it. One of my friends' husbands joked, "I'm not too worried about my sex life. I know I'll have sex again in a few months. I just hope it will be with my wife."

I have heard that there are some of you out there who can't wait to have sex again, but I've never talked to one of you in the flesh and blood, so I'm not convinced that isn't just a rumor started by men to encourage us to have sex before we're ready. If you are living proof that sex after pregnancy is an anticipated, joyous event, please write or e-mail me so that I'll know you exist.

If you are not one of these rumored sex fiends, take it slow, relax, and start with intimacy before intercourse. Cuddle in bed together, take a bath together, massage each other, or light some candles and explore each other's body again. Then, with a lubricant in hand (and maybe a good stiff drink in the other), give it a try. Sex may be painful at first, but it will get better. Each time, the newly repaired tissue will toughen up and your inhibitions will loosen up. If the pain, dryness, and fear persist, make an appointment with your doctor.

A recent survey found that over half of us are embarrassed to bring up sex difficulties with our doctors. Our mothers' generation was supposed to be embarrassed by sex, not ours. Talk to your doctor and talk to your friends, they'll tell you that postpartum sex difficulties are common and completely normal—and validation may be just what you need to give it another try tonight and overcome the stress associated with sex.

Don't Stress Out Your Fat Cells

After six weeks of baby euphoria and new mother bliss, you may have thought that when the stork brought your baby, she bundled up your stress and whisked it away for good. Don't we wish. If the stressful reality of your "harried with children" life hasn't hit yet, prepare yourself. It can knock you over like a palm tree in a hurricane. All of a sudden, the wave of tension engulfs you as it becomes quite clear that you're not only responsible for your baby, but everyone and everything else again. Your baby's diapers need to be changed, and so do the beds. Your baby needs to be washed, and so do the floors. Your baby needs to be fed, and so does the rest of the family. Your baby needs to be comforted, and so does your husband. Your baby's hospital bills need to be paid, and so do the other bills. The list goes on and on. Sure, you were stressed from a demanding workload before having a child, but now those prebaby days seem more like summer camp. You used to do about eighteen hours of housework a week; now it will almost double to thirty-three hours a week. You used to have at least forty-five minutes a day to relax; now you're lucky if you get five uninterrupted minutes of solitude. And that's on a good day.

Not coincidentally, the stress of motherhood starts to bubble and boil right when your endorphin rush is wearing off and your outside help is quickly diminishing. All of a sudden you realize that your mother has gone home, your friends have stopped coming by, your husband has gone back to his hectic work schedule, and you're all alone. The University of Minnesota found that outside help between month one and month three dropped by 33 percent. Have you started to notice the absence of casserole dishes left on your doorstep? Fewer phone calls offering assistance? Fewer visits by family and friends to help with cleaning, cooking, and child care?

Whenever you're feeling undersupported, overwhelmed, and overstressed, every single cell in your body is stressing out with you. Your heart cells tense up, and your heart rate and blood pressure rise. Your lung cells get overanxious, and your breathing increases. Your stomach cells get overstimulated, and they oversecrete stomach acids. Your skin cells constrict, and they are deprived of oxygen and nutrients. And your fat cells freak out, and they respond by storing more and growing larger. Cortisol, one of the stress hormones, has been found to stimulate fat storage, especially in the abdominal area. So, too much stress not only prevents you from enjoying your baby and your life, it also prevents your body from losing weight and stomach from flattening out.

Some stress, of course, is inevitable, and some worries are unavoidable. Take the universal concern every new mother has about the health and well-being of her baby. It works in our favor, keeping us alert and tuned in to our baby's needs. But other worries of motherhood are a waste of energy. For example, are you worried about being a good mother? If you love and care for your baby, you're a good mother. Period. End of discussion. There are many different parenting styles, and there will always be skills to work on. Or, are you like Janet, who was obsessively worried that she would become her mother? She was so intent upon doing the opposite of everything her mother did, that one day she stormed into my office with a startling revelation—she was trying so hard not to become her mother that she woke up that morning realizing that she had become her father instead. The horror!

What's your biggest stress-producing worry right now? For three out of every four of us postpartum women, it's our weight. And what do we do when we're worried about our weight? We increase our stress level by getting on the scale and trying on our prepregnancy clothes. We know that we weigh more than we want to right now, but we hop on that stress-inducing, body-image zapping device just to torture ourselves. And if we make the mistake of weighing ourselves before we've breastfed, those milk-filled mammaries can tip the scale up an additional two pounds, and we tip over the edge of sanity. Trust me. The scale is not your friend. Remove it from your life, and you'll be removing some unnecessary stress.

You might as well stay clear of your closet, too. We know those prepregnancy clothes won't fit, but we struggle to get them past our thighs and over our hips, only to rip them in the fight or look like a stuffed sausage whose casing is too small. And if you try to wear something out in public just to prove to yourself that you can fit into your "skinny clothes," everyone will know you're wearing an outfit that is two sizes too small and will whisper behind your back that you've "let yourself go and are too cheap to buy new clothes." Don't let a clothes crisis catapult you into the stress ionosphere. Save yourself the unnecessary strain, and restrain yourself from the closet. Go out and buy yourself a new outfit (nonmaternity, of course) that fits comfortably instead. When the going gets tough, the tough go shopping. Retail therapy may be the most effective stress therapy there is.

But, of course, shopping isn't the only technique you can use to silence your stress and relax your fat cells. Nor may it be the most feasible. If you have other children at home, you may not have a spare minute to run to the mall for some retail therapy—or run to the masseuse or manicurist or meditation workshop for some intensive stress reduction. Between infant care, toddler care, and child care, plus housework, homework, and paperwork, it may be ten years before you have enough "free time" in your schedule to effectively combat stress. So, it's best to start right now with some practical tips to tame the tension; techniques you can use today with an infant at home, tomorrow with a carload of kids, and every day with an overbooked schedule. I call these practical tips "Stress Busters," and here are ten designed specifically for mothers:

- **Stress Buster #1: Experience the joy of not cooking.** Personally, I've never found joy in cooking. If you did, you'll be too distracted to enjoy it now with crying babies, fighting siblings, and the "witching hour." So take time out from kitchen chaos and supper stress with take-out food or quality frozen dinners.

- **Stress Buster #2: Fake a smile.** Even if a frown is permanently pasted to your face, force the corners of your mouth to turn up, and you'll immediately turn down your stress response. Or better yet, show your pearly whites with a genuine smile. Smiling, even a fake one, releases relaxing brain chemicals, and you don't even have to leave your home to take advantage of it. Sometimes nothing is funnier than what innocently comes out of your children's mouths. One of my clients shared a discussion she was having with her five-year-old son, explaining the importance of doing well in school to get ahead in life, when he interrupted, "But Mom, I already have a head."

- **Stress Buster #3: Have a girls' night out.** After being cooped up in the house for the last couple of months, you could probably use one. According to UCLA researchers, stressed out men run away and isolate themselves in front of the TV, whereas stressed out women run over to a friend's house and surround themselves with female energy. Our stress hormones automatically decrease when we're in the presence of other women.

- **Stress Buster #4: Phone a friend (it's one of your lifelines).** If you can't be with your girlfriends, the next best thing is to hear their voices. You can talk about nothing in particular or everything that's stressing you out. Sometimes just venting, screaming, or crying to a sympathetic ear is all it takes to feel the tension lift.

- **Stress Buster #5: Buy wash and wear.** Forget dry cleaning and ironing; wash and wear will save you time and money as well as your sanity. Haven't you heard what "freedom of the press" means for women? No-iron clothes.

- **Stress Buster #6: Stock up on paper plates (and cups and napkins and towels).** With fewer dishes to wash, few dishes to potentially break, and fewer dishes to put away, you'll be glad you stocked up on paper. And be sure to recycle so you won't put too much stress on the environment, either.

- **Stress Buster #7: Say thank you, don't write it.** I remember the stress I felt from the growing number of thank-you notes that I still hadn't written. When a friend told me, "Just thank me now and forget the note," I was overjoyed with relief. In fact, it felt so good that I started taking the initiative by asking, "Can I verbally thank you now instead of sending a note?"

- **Stress Buster #8: Have the babysitter come one-half hour early.** When you're going out for a romantic dinner, relaxing movie, or festive party, don't get stressed out before you go out. Have the sitter hold down the fort and feed the troops while you take your time getting ready.

- **Stress Buster #9: Let the house get dirty (for a day).** A messy house stresses me out, too, but one day won't make much of a difference. If you took the time to clean up, it will look like you did nothing by the end of the day anyway. So release the stressful chore for a day. Your baby won't notice, your other kids won't care, and your husband, well, he can pitch in or call a cleaning service if he doesn't like it. After Karen tried the "dirty house for a day" approach, she was forever hooked and dubbed herself Mrs. Unclean, saying, "If cleanliness really is next to godliness, I'm going straight to hell—but at least I'll be relaxed when I get there."

- **Stress Buster #10: Don't get mad, get Dad.** A recent poll of thirty thousand couples found that women are the more stressed of the pair. No surprise, but the researchers also found that mothers were 50 percent more likely than fathers to be "in a bad mood" from too much stress. Don't let your stress cause anger and hostility; call upon Dad to help lighten the load.

But don't just call upon Dad for support and a helping hand—call anyone and everyone you can to help you destress, relax your fat cells, and ease into your new role of mother.

Beg, Borrow, and Steal: Getting All the Support You Need

With your stress level building and your outside support dwindling, it's now up to you to seek out the support you need—from your partner, family, and friends. Let's talk about your partner first. To elicit his support, you need to verbally ask for it by speaking slowly, clearly, and specifically. If you don't ask, and instead expect him to enthusiastically volunteer for the exact task you need done, you'll be waiting all night with growing disappointment and frustration. He'll come home from work, open a beer, grab the remote control (which, by the way, was just identified as the most vital device in a man's life), and superglue himself to the couch.

It's not that men purposely ignore our needs, it's that they are unable to read our facial expressions and body language. Research has actually proven this. They look at us, but they don't register the bags under our eyes, our dragging feet, our unwashed hair, our dry, flaking skin, or our callused hands. So, we have no choice but to take matters into our own hands, point out our harried state of disrepair, and ask for exactly what we need before the beer and remote control set the tone for the evening. And if at first we don't receive—ask, ask again. Repeating yourself is necessary because men really do listen with only half a brain. Research has actually proven this, too. Indiana University School of Medicine discovered that men only use the left half of their brain while listening (we, on the other hand, use both halves), which explains why one request is never quite enough—and why you may have to repeatedly ask your spouse to help with the housework, pick up dinner on the way home, put the baby to bed, bathe the other kids, or take care of all the kids while you go out for that much-needed girls' night out, shopping spree, or day to yourself.

"Not my husband!" protested Maya. "If I ask enough times, he may eventually listen, but I could never leave him with the kids. He couldn't handle it. The house would be a total mess, the baby would be starving and filthy, and the TV would be on all day. I really don't think he'd survive." That's many a new mother's reaction to leaving the baby and kids with Dad. Of course, we're better at child care than they are—we're mothers. But they may be better than we think, and the more they do it, the better they'll get. Plus, children need alone time with their fathers, and we need alone time with ourselves. They may not care for the little ones like we would or like we'd want them to, but they will survive.

Maya still had a hard time believing that her husband, or any man for that matter, could play Mr. Mom, so the next day she sent me an e-mail to drive her point home. It was an idea for the next *Survivor* TV show, which I took the liberty of improving on some, but it would be a guaranteed success among skeptical female viewers.

> Twelve men will each be dropped off in an unidentified suburb with a minivan, four kids, and no access to fast food. They must keep the house clean, keep the kids clean, correct all homework, cook nutritious meals, plan birthday parties for all

> the kids, and attend PTA meetings and parent–teacher conferences. Their competitions will include cleaning up after a sick child at 3 A.M., dealing with a temper tantrum while in line at the grocery store, potty training a three-year-old, getting a four-year-old to eat peas, remembering all the relatives' birthdays, and figuring out how to get all four children to soccer games at different but overlapping times and be there to watch each one of them. The kids get to vote them off. The winner gets to go back to his job.

At least the Internet is good for a few laughs. I replied back to Maya, "Point taken. So, maybe we don't take off for a week, but as long as we leave them with a stocked refrigerator on a day that they don't have to leave the house, they should be able to 'survive' for at least a few hours."

What if you don't have a significant other to ask for child care or home care support (or one that is unresponsive to your needs)? Turn to your girlfriends and female relatives. You'll only have to ask once, and the results may be a good deal more rewarding—you get to connect with other women who understand what you're going through. Ask them to pick up a few things from the grocery store for you, to take your baby for a walk, to take your older kids to the park, to pick up your daughter from school, or to organize a girls' night out.

But even your friends and family won't know that you need help unless you ask for it. If you don't ask, there's a good chance they'll automatically assume that you're doing just fine on your own. This is what happened in my situation. I made the mistake of not asking, which only made everyone think, "Deb's doing great." And I was great. But I still needed help. It took me weeks before I let my female circle know that I still needed them, and when I did, it made all the difference in the world. They were thrilled to pitch in and help, and I was thrilled to be helped by people that I loved. *All you need to do is ask, and I recommend asking sooner rather than later.*

What if there is absolutely no one to ask? Clare was a single mother of a six-year-old son who was transferred a thousand miles away from her family and friends right before her second baby was born. Since there was no one she could call to ask for help, she quickly had to find a support system. While still on maternity leave, she hired a neighborhood teenager to come over in the afternoons, joined a Mommy and Me class, took her baby to Gymboree, and frequented the local coffee shop—where she found dozens of other new mothers with babies in tow who were just as eager for companionship and support.

She also discovered that *she* was an important component of her support system, and the best support she could give herself was to take the pressure off to "get everything done." When she first came to see me, she was feeling unproductive and unorganized with her growing list of things to do, so I had her do an activity that highlighted her highly productive daily accomplishments. I had her write down everything she did in one day. Here is her list:

I breastfed my baby
Woke up my first grader
Made him breakfast
Packed his lunch
Got him dressed
Walked him to the bus stop
Breastfed again
Put my baby down for a nap
Returned five phone calls
Did three loads of laundry
Gave my baby a bath
Got her dressed
Breastfed again
Went to the grocery store
Picked up the dry cleaning
Got the car washed
Breastfed again

Put her down for a nap
Had lunch
Folded the laundry
Paid some bills
Returned more phone calls
Breastfed again
Walked to the bus stop to meet my son
Made him a snack
Put my baby down for another nap
Played cards with my son
Got dinner ready
Called my mother
Breastfed again
Ate dinner with my son
Gave him a bubble bath
Read him a book
Put him to bed
Breastfed again
Cleaned the kitchen
Vacuumed the rug
E-mailed friends
Wrote a dozen thank-you notes
Breastfed again
Collapsed in bed

Could Clare have accomplished any more? Could you have accomplished any more today? Not without a live-in nanny, a hired chef, and a personal assistant. But there is something missing from many of our lists: *us*. Where are our bubble baths? Our snacks? Our playtime? Our nap time? Our bedtime reading? Including just one pampering activity a day is giving ourselves the gift of personal support. So, be kind to yourself by taking the pressure off and taking a nap or bath instead. You're getting everything done that needs to be done. And right now, that's all that really matters.

What's Your Postpartum Peace Plan for the Next Six Weeks?

After nurturing yourself and letting others nurture you back to health for the last six weeks, it's time to take your first step in outsmarting your postpartum fat cells by making some specific changes in the way you move and feed your body. So what's your plan? Which recommendations hit home with you, what made sense for your new lifestyle, and how will you make peace with your fat cells? Check all that apply.

What Will You Do to Pamper Yourself?

____ I will realize that my body is still in the midst of repair and continues to need rest and care.

____ I will form my own support system with other new mothers, babysitters, and mother–baby groups.

____ I will put myself on my daily to-do list, adding a pampering activity that will make me feel good.

What Will You Do to Eat With a Regular Meal Schedule?

____ I will identify the eating habits formed in pregnancy that are working against my postpartum weight-loss efforts.

____ I will put my portions in proportion by acknowledging how small a standard serving really is.

____ I will eyeball a small portion first, and eat second.

____ I will read nutrition labels to see how many portions are in the bag or box.

____ I will use my hand to define the size of a small meal.

____ I will focus on how much I'm eating, not what I'm eating.

What Will You Do to Actively Move Your Body?

____ I will start moving my body slowly and stop if my body (or my baby) tells me that I'm doing too much too soon.

____ I will think before I move by formulating a realistic plan I can stick with.

____ I will take walks with my baby whenever I can.

____ I will fidget whenever possible by getting up, pacing around the room, and walking around the house.

____ I will move my body anytime I can—with the goal of having my movement add up to thirty or more minutes a day.

____ I will find my exercise motivator to keep me moving.

What Will You Do to Calm Your Stress?

____ I will let go of worries that are a waste of energy.

____ I will relax about my weight, knowing that the more relaxed I am, the more weight I'll lose.

____ I will not get on the scale or try on my prepregnancy clothes.

____ I will specifically ask for exactly what I need—and if at first I don't receive, I'll ask, ask again.

____ I will practice some or all of the ten stress busters by smiling, going out with the girls, letting the house get dirty, or buying paper plates.

What Will You Do to Embrace Your New Body?

____ I will give my body time to lose weight on its own schedule; and realize that these next six weeks are not my body's chosen time to burn fat.

____ I will go out and buy myself a new outfit that fits well and that I feel good in.

____ I will let my partner see me naked with the lights on.

____ I will realize that it is normal to have the sex jitters and that the pain and fear will subside over time.

____ I will give my body intimacy with bubble baths, hugs, cuddling, massage, and foreplay.

Chapter Six

The Next Six Months: Out, Out, Damn Fat

Three months have passed since you delivered your baby—short months when you think of your baby's changes, and excruciatingly long months when you take inventory of your body's changes. Your baby is smiling at you already, but you're frowning over your still-overweight body. Your baby has rolled over for the first time, but your weight hasn't gone much of anywhere. Your baby is reaching up and touching your face, but your body satisfaction is spiraling down, and you're grabbing at your stomach, wondering if you'll *ever* lose this pregnancy weight.

You will—and this is the time to do it. Up until now, your body wouldn't let you lose a significant amount of weight: Your body was recovering, your breast milk was coming in, and your fat cells were in the rest mode, saving their stored fat for a possible famine. During the next six months or so, your fat cells *will* release fat, your stomach and thighs *will* shrink, and your body *will* lose the pregnancy weight, as long as you take advantage of this opportune time to outsmart your postpartum fat cells by making some simple and effective changes in the way you think, eat, and move.

Are you ready for these next six months? Of course you're ready; you've been ready to lose weight since day one. But are you excited about the process? Are you motivated to help your body with moderate eating and regular exercise? Do you believe you can lose the weight and regain your shape? Believing you can do it is half the battle. To assess your readiness, motivation, and belief system, take a moment to answer these three questions:

1. Do you wake up in the morning feeling excited to take on another potential fat-burning day?
2. Are you confident of your body's ability to lose weight?
3. When you think of the future, can you picture yourself fit, trim, and healthy?

Joann didn't hesitate before answering an emphatic "No! No! and No! Every morning I wake up with a doom-and-gloom feeling, disgusted with my body and completely discouraged about another day without weight loss. And when I think about the future, I can picture myself quite clearly all right, but I'm a cross between the Michelin Man and the Pillsbury Doughboy. Even with regular exercise and healthy eating, I know that I'll never get this weight off."

Unfortunately, Joann's reaction is all too common. When I surveyed postpartum women, the vast majority felt negatively about their bodies, their ability to lose weight, and their future weight loss. But negative thinking may very well lead to a negative outcome. If we think that we'll never lose the weight, it may become a self-fulfilling prophecy. We'll set ourselves up to stay overweight by overeating in frustration, coming up with every excuse not to exercise, and then saying, "See, I knew I wouldn't be able to lose the weight." Your body won't lose the weight if your mind won't let it. It's what I call the You Are What You Think Effect—what you think affects your fat cells. If you are thinking that "it will be a cold day in hell before I lose weight," your fat cells will say, "Okay, fine by us, we don't mind waiting until hell freezes over before we release any fat." But if, instead, you are thinking that "I can do this. I'm an intelligent woman who has the patience to lose weight in a healthy way," your fat cells will say, "Well, okay, she's the boss. We can't argue with her slow and healthy approach. Count us in."

Focus the mind and the body will follow; positive thinking will lead to a positive outcome. So positive, that a recent study from the Mayo Clinic found that optimists live longer than pessimists. The researchers followed both personality types for three decades, and discovered that the optimists were 19 percent less likely to die early. They believed they could stay healthy, sought solutions to wellness, and were rewarded with a positive outcome. You can be a long-living, healthy, lean optimist too. *If you start to believe you can lose the weight, you'll be motivated to make the necessary changes in your lifestyle to lead you to that outcome.*

When I shared this research with Joann and encouraged her to start thinking positively about her weight loss, she quickly replied, "Oh, I can be positive all right. . . . I'm absolutely, 100 percent positive that I'll never get this weight off!" Not quite the response I was looking for, but nonetheless, I appreciated her sense of humor. No matter what you're feeling right now about your future weight loss, a sense of humor and ability to laugh at yourself are vital to your success—because the next 180 days or so are your knock-down-drag-out days to outsmart your postpartum fat cells. Laughter will not only keep your spirits high when your energy and motivation are low, it will also boost your metabolism, strengthen your abdominal muscles, and shrink your fat cells. A burst of laughter can electrify your body with energy. The contagious giggles can constrict your stomach muscles so tightly that the pain leaves you doubled over on the floor yelling, "Stop!" Going to a comedy show can burn hundreds of fat calories, and if the comedian is really good, you could burn more calories than going to the gym. So, laugh freely and often, because if you try to suppress it, it will only go back down and spread to your hips.

This chapter, like all the others, will be sprinkled with humor in an attempt to prevent hip expansion and promote fat-cell shrinkage. It will also provide the serious science to give you all the research and skills to successfully outsmart your postpartum fat cells. But the underlying theme will be positive thinking—to help you become more optimistic about your postpartum weight loss, eating, exercising, and female body.

Thinking positively about your postpartum body may not be an easy task. You may have had a negative body image since puberty, and now, since pregnancy, it has sunk into a black hole. But in order to lose weight, you have to accept your body and improve your body image first. We've been led to believe that it's the other way around; that weight loss leads to body acceptance. It doesn't. Thinner women are just as dissatisfied with their bodies as larger women, and weight loss doesn't occur until after you accept your body. Stanford University School of Medicine researchers found that those women who were happiest with their bodies before trying to lose weight were twice as likely to shed excess pounds as those who were dissatisfied with their bodies—*proving beyond a shadow of a doubt that the best weight-loss program is a body-acceptance program.* When you accept and respect your body, you're more likely to keep it active and feed it moderately.

Are you ready to accept your postpartum body with open arms? Are you ready to fall in love with your love handles? Serenade your stretch marks? Whisper sweet nothings to your waist? Get weak in the knees over your thighs? I may be pushing it a bit too far, but I encourage you to keep an open mind. After you spend some time on body acceptance, you never know, you just might decide you want to get pregnant all over again just so you can fall in love with your postpartum body a second time.

Twenty-Five Ways to Love Your Postpartum Body

"You've got to be kidding! You expect me to love this fat, jiggly postpartum body? I don't think so. Loathe is more like it. I wake up every day disgusted with the way I look and go to bed every night detesting my rolls of fat. I refuse to wear shorts or sleeveless tops, my lingerie is in permanent storage, and I wouldn't be caught dead in a bathing suit if you paid me a million dollars. I won't even have any pictures taken of my baby and me. The sight of my blubbery body is just too much to handle."

Here's Joann again—our postpartum pessimist who had one of the strongest negative reactions to body acceptance that I've ever come across. Instead of trying to convince her that she could love her body just the way it is, I asked her to do a little guided imagery. To close her eyes and just imagine what would happen to her life if she woke up tomorrow liking her body. Here's her report: "I woke up smiling. I went to the mirror and actually smiled at the sight of my body, something I haven't done since I was nine years old. Then I took a long bath with my baby, something I've never done because I don't want anyone, including an infant with blurred vision, to see my body naked. Then I went to lunch with some friends and their babies and ordered a pepperoni pizza instead of a salad, something I haven't done since I started my first diet at age sixteen. Then I went swimming in our neighborhood pool, something I haven't done since before I got pregnant. And then for the finale, I surprised my husband with a romantic evening once our baby was in bed (in your imagination, babies can go to bed early and stay there)—a candlelight dinner, a little wine, some dancing, and then on to marathon sex. And when we were done, I didn't even back away from the bed to prevent him from seeing the cellulite on the back of my thighs. Now that's something I haven't done since our honeymoon!"

By doing this activity, Joann realized that her body dissatisfaction made her miss out on the joys of life and that she had been putting her life on hold and wasting valuable time with her baby, husband, and friends. She had much joy to gain (and weight to lose) by working on body acceptance. And so do you. Imagine how your life would change if you woke up tomorrow liking your body—then use the following Twenty-five Ways to Love Your Postpartum Body as your tools for getting there in real life. Some of the recommendations are tongue-in-cheek, and some are dead serious—but they will all help you to view your body in a more accepting light, and therefore, make you a lighter postpartum woman.

1. **Look at a picture of yourself when you were nine months' pregnant.** You're a fraction of the size you were three months ago, and that will help you appreciate how much weight you've already lost and how much your body has already changed.
2. **Take a bath with your baby.** Babies love the feel of our naked bodies, and if they think your body is warm, nurturing, cuddly, and beautiful—you can too.
3. **Don't have a fit, get fit.** According to a recent study from London, women who exercise have a higher self-image than those who don't. No surprise, but you may think their body acceptance was due to the fact that they must be thinner (after all, they do exercise). Not so. They weighed an average of twelve pounds more than the sedentary women studied, but they were stronger, fitter, and more confident.
4. **Lift your image.** Women who lift weights three times a week experience an even greater increase in self-image than those who walk (or do other aerobic exercise) three times a week. Build muscle, and you'll build a better body image. Or better yet—do both—lift weights and walk and you'll double the body-image benefits.
5. **Go out and buy a new outfit.** It's rated as the number one quick fix for a bad body day. You've probably been wearing the same black stretch pants day-in and day-out and could use a little wardrobe lift with retail therapy. Shopping not only reduces stress, it also increases self-esteem.

6. **Listen to music, don't watch it.** The *International Journal of Obesity* recently published a study showing that music videos did more damage to our body image than any other television show (maybe MTV really means "Many Thin Vixens"). What shows boosted our body confidence? Anything on a sports channel, which may explain why men feel better about their bodies regardless of their weights. They know a little body image secret: You don't even have to play sports; just watching other people get fit works to improve your self-image.
7. **Have an out-of-body experience.** Many of us have what's called "body distortion"; we see our bodies as bigger than they actually are. The University of Florida found that the typical woman overestimates her body size by 25 percent. No wonder one hundred million women wake up every morning feeling fat—we erroneously think we are. Next time you look in the mirror, step out of your body for a moment and look at it accurately. Your thighs are not so big that they thunder when you walk; they may chafe, but they don't clap. Your stomach is not the size of Texas; Houston maybe, but not the whole state. Your body is not obese; it may be bigger than you'd like, but it's 25 percent smaller than you think.
8. **Hold your head high.** Your posture can put you in a position of confidence. Stand straight and tall, and you'll feel straight and tall. Slouch, and your stomach will pouch out even more. Try it right now and see if you can feel the difference.
9. **Talk back.** When that inner critic in your head tells you that you're "fat and worthless," don't listen. Tell it to "shut the @#*& up." You're not fat; you're a postpartum woman who just had a baby. And you're certainly not worthless; just ask your baby.
10. **Initiate Sex.** Not only will you get a kick out of your husband's surprised and longing reaction, you'll kick up your self-esteem; 38 percent of us say that initiating sex boosts our body image.
11. **Give someone a body compliment.** Stop a stranger on the street and say, "That outfit looks great on you" or tell a friend, "I love your full figure" or "You have gorgeous legs." You may risk

her thinking that you're trying to pick her up, but it's her body image that will be picked up—and yours will too. The giver feels just as good as the receiver.

12. **Give yourself a body compliment.** The typical woman averages eighteen critical comments a day. We wake up saying we feel fat, we go through the day reminding ourselves how fat we are, and we go to bed telling ourselves that we'll get even fatter while we sleep. Pick a day and start it with a body compliment—"I love my big, full breasts" or "Look at these beautiful long legs"—and you'll end the day feeling more body confident.
13. **Accept body compliments from others.** When someone tells you that you look great, what do you do? Most women deny the compliment in some self-deprecating way. Instead of saying, "No I don't; I still have twenty more pounds to lose," try "Thank you; I'm getting there."
14. **Tell people you have calliopygia.** Some may think you have a rare, contagious disease, but what you're really telling them is that you have a very attractive derriere. It's Latin, meaning "beautiful buttocks," and thousands of years ago when this word first originated, the bigger the buttocks, the more beautiful the bottom.
15. **Volunteer to be a nude model in an art class.** I'm serious. It may be just the body therapy you need. The Real Woman Project has been using this body-image booster for years and has received national attention for its positive results. After women pose and see the finished product, they are more likely to view their bodies as a work of art.
16. **Go to an art museum.** If you won't strip down to your birthday suit to model, the next best thing is to go and see works of art. When you see the Rubenesque figures lounging in a meadow, feasting on a meal, or breastfeeding their babies, you'll realize that soft curves, ample thighs, and a voluptuous body really are beautiful.
17. **Dye your hair red.** Think blondes have more fun? Think again. When self-confidence is rated based on hair color, redheads top

the list, followed by brunettes, and last on the list is blondes. When you have the time to get your hair done again, you may want to consider going red for your self-esteem.

18. **Move to Samoa.** Because Samoans associate fat with health and wealth, a size sixteen is actually considered petite. The typical Samoan mother stands 5'5", weighs two hundred pounds, and is proud of it.
19. **Buy *Mode* magazine.** Relatively new on the stands, *Mode* is the only fashion magazine that should make it into the hands of postpartum women. Instead of emaciated models wearing a size two, you'll find real, well-fed, well-proportioned, regular-sized women wearing a size fourteen, who are old enough to have borne children themselves.
20. **Become an advocate for body acceptance.** Join a grassroots organization such as Body Positive, the National Association to Advance Fat Acceptance, or WINS (We Insist on Natural Shapes). Write letters to fashion magazines and television networks condemning the thin ideal (or condoning their rise above it), share your views with other women in your community, and help girls and teens respect the bodies they were born with.
21. **Find five things you like about your body.** They're there, they're just buried beneath the body parts you don't like (i.e., your stomach, hips, and thighs). I don't care what they are—your little toe, your eyebrows, your birthmark, or the nape of your neck—I just care that you acknowledge them every day.
22. **Throw your body a surprise party.** Invite the bubble bath, facial mask, scented lotion, loofah sponge, aromatic candles, and relaxing music. Then surprise your body at nine o'clock sharp—and don't be late.
23. **Put together a body image repair kit and give it to a friend.** Include bath products, a gift certificate for a massage, a copy of *Mode* magazine, the definition of calliopygia, and you might want to throw in a bottle of wine because everything seems to look better when you're a little tipsy.

24. **If you must, give yourself five minutes of body-bashing time.** Set the timer, knock yourself out, then let go of any bad body thoughts for the rest of the day.
25. **Take the road less traveled.** Picture yourself at a fork in the road. One way leads you to body acceptance; the other to continued body hatred. Which will you choose? Joann answered, "Neither. When I picture a fork in the road, all I want to do is pick it up and walk across the street to Denny's."

Let's try that last one again. Picture yourself at a fork in the road. One way leads you to a healthy relationship with your body where feeling beautiful is more important than looking beautiful; the other leads you to an unhealthy relationship where the size of your body is more important than the size of your heart. Which will you choose? Good. We'll journey on that road to body acceptance together. There may be a few bumps and potholes along the way, but you won't regret it. You'll be a healthier, happier, fitter, and trimmer woman who respects her body morning, noon, and night. If you continue down the path of body dissatisfaction, you certainly won't be happy, and it's doubtful you'll be healthy, fit, or trim either. When you dislike your body, you don't respect it enough to treat it well with food, fitness, and everything else that makes you feel good.

Your Five Fat-Burning, Metabolism-Boosting, Muscle-Building, Stomach-Flattening Guidelines

The three-month grace period is over. The "go easy, take it slow, do just a few minutes" exercise recommendation from the last chapter is history. It's time to blast away postpartum fat—and exercise is your dynamite. After resting peacefully for the last ninety days, it will take something like an explosion of exercise to get your fat cells up, alert, and ready to release fat.

Try to visualize the fat-exploding effects of exercise. Your fat cells are half-dozing in recliners when all of a sudden, they are ejected out of their chairs with a frightening shock. "Hey, she's not just strolling her baby around the block, she's power walking with a baby jogger on a hiking trail that's a three-mile loop. But maybe she's just walking up to that clearing to meet a friend for a picnic. Maybe her baby will start crying, and she'll have to stop and breastfeed. Maybe she'll trip over that tree stump up ahead and twist her ankle. Wishful thinking. We're past the picnic tables and tree stump already, her baby's sound asleep, and she's picked up the pace even more. Damn. She must be reading one of those 'Outsmarting Us' books. We haven't had to do anything but store and rest for the past twelve months, and now she's issuing us a work order for double shifts. Sound the horn, round up the troops, start punching the clock—it's time to activate our fat-releasing enzymes and provide the 350 calories she needs for her aerobic walk. But she'd better not do this again tomorrow. After this much work, I'm going to need a day off to rest."

With exercise, your fat cells get a new job description. They don't just store, grow, and rest—they release, shrink, and work to make you a smaller postpartum woman. But to ignite your fat cells and train them in the art of fat burning, you have to exercise in a certain way. *It has to be aerobic for approximately forty-five minutes at a moderate intensity three to five times a week—with some stomach crunches and weight training thrown in.* Before you start telling me that you don't have the time (I already know you don't), let me explain why it's vital to somehow, someway make the time by sharing the rationale behind the five fat-burning, metabolism-boosting, muscle-building, stomach-flattening guidelines.

#1 Exercise Aerobically

Aerobic exercise is the *only* way to get your fat cells working and releasing. As you probably know, aerobic exercise includes walking, running, cycling, swimming, rowing, stair climbing, cross-country skiing, or any other activity that uses your major muscle groups, your buttocks and thighs, in a rhythmical nonstop movement. *Nonstop* is a key word in the definition. In order for your fat cells to manufacture the fat-releasing enzymes and dump fat out into your bloodstream to fuel your muscles—you have to convince them that it's absolutely necessary. You need to make it crystal clear that you need some of their fat, and nonstop is the argument that wins them over. They won't respond if you keep stopping to rest, tie your shoes, gaze at a vista point, or run into a store for an errand. They'll think that you can do it just fine without their help; you have plenty of glucose hanging around to fuel your muscles and get the job done. So, they'll yawn, roll over, and go back to sleep. This nonstop argument is also the reason why such stop-start activities such as golf, tennis, racquetball, softball, yoga, and weight lifting aren't fat-burning. Not that these activities are worthless—to the contrary, they will boost your metabolism and tone your muscles—but they won't burn fat.

#2 Go the Distance

A walk around the block won't whittle away fat. A run up the stairs won't stir your fat cells. A bike ride down the street won't release fat. They may be nonstop, but they're not long enough. You have to go the distance to outsmart your postpartum fat cells—whatever distance you can accomplish in about forty-five minutes.

"Forty-five minutes? What about the twenty- to thirty-minute recommendation I've heard over and over again?" asked Janice, who was doing thirty minutes and wondering why she wasn't seeing a change in her body. Twenty to thirty minutes works great for men (who were born with the fat-burning machinery to release fat quickly and efficiently) and teenage girls (whose bodies haven't yet geared up for pregnancy). But for us postadolescent, postpartum females, twenty to thirty minutes is just when our fat cells start to find exercise interesting. The older we get, the bolder our fat cells get—refusing to budge for any aerobic exercise less than thirty minutes.

Every minute after thirty minutes is a fat-burning minute—that's when our fat cells activate the fat-releasing enzymes and shrink. And when you work up to forty-five minutes, you'll get a full fifteen minutes of fat burning time. A recent study showed just how powerful that forty-five minutes can be. Those postpartum women who didn't exercise only lost one-and-a-half pounds in ten weeks, but those who moved their bodies aerobically for forty-five minutes four times a week lost over ten pounds. Now that's what I call powerful—and motivating! So motivating that I hope it will encourage you to somehow, some way find three or four blocks of forty-five minutes each week to exercise away that pregnancy fat. Of everything I'll share in this book, exercise is the #1 fat-cell outsmarter, because it changes the way your fat cells function, teaching them that they aren't just storage receptacles, but shrinking machines.

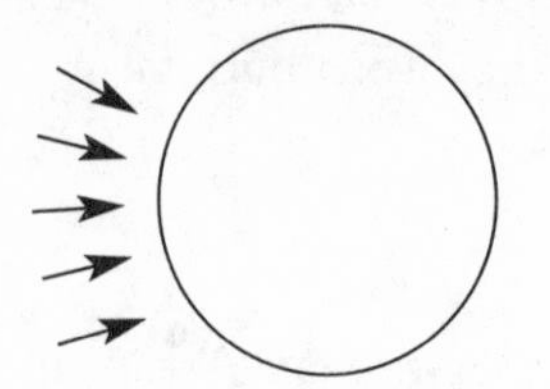

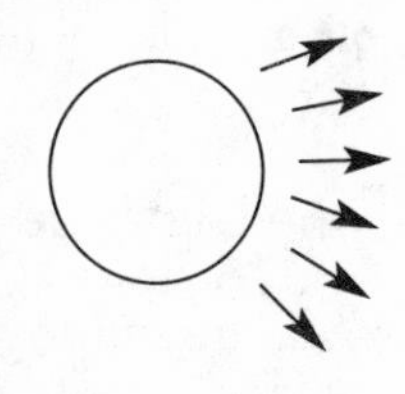

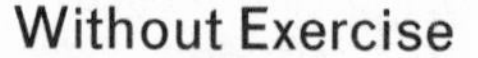

Without Exercise

With Forty-five minutes of Aerobic Exercise Three to Five Times a Week

"But I can't do forty-five minutes," complained Natalie. "I've blocked out the time to do it by walking with my baby or trading babysitting time with a friend. But within twenty minutes I conk out and can barely take another step." At the beginning of your exercise program, you're not conditioned enough to be able to go for forty-five minutes, so slowly build up your duration by adding five-minute increments every week or two. But Natalie's inability to go forty-five minutes wasn't from a lack of conditioning. It was because she was over-exhausting herself by exercising at too high an intensity, thinking that the harder she pushed herself, the more fat she'd burn.

#3 Pace Yourself

The intensity of your exercise, or how hard and fast you move your body, is another vital guideline for fat release. You want to go at a good enough pace to increase your heart rate and breathing, but if you are huffing and puffing and pushing yourself to the point of exertion, the exercise becomes anaerobic (meaning without oxygen). You can't get enough oxygen into your body to stimulate fat release no matter how hard you try. "Aerobic" exercise means "with oxygen," and you have to have a ready supply of oxygen to release fat. When you're out of breath, it means that your breathing can't meet the oxygen demands of your body. And if you can't meet the oxygen demands of your body, you're exercising anaerobically and can't burn fat.

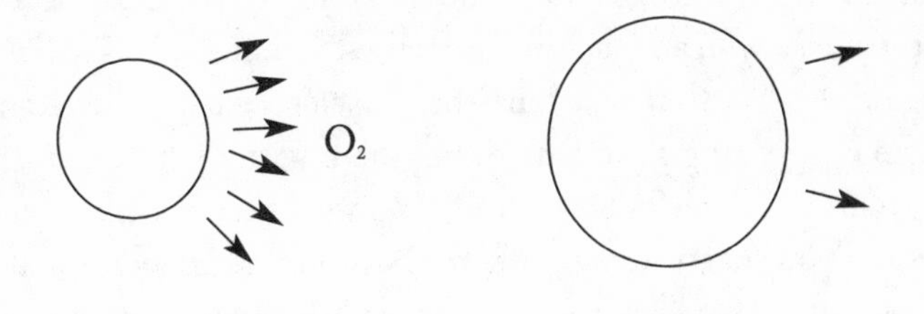

With Oxygen Without Oxygen

How do you know you're exercising at the right intensity? By monitoring your rate of breathing—you want it to be increased, but not to the point of hyperventilating. And the best way to check out your breathing is to do the "talk test." If you can't talk, you're working too hard. If you can recite the whole Declaration of Independence, you're not working hard enough. But if you can complete a three or four word sentence before needing to take a breath, you're working at a perfect intensity.

Slow down your pace, make sure you can talk, go a longer distance that lasts forty-five minutes, and do it three to five times a week, *and your fat cells will shrink.* The only caveat is that they may be a bit selective about where they shrink. The fat cells in your thighs will shrink (hooray!), as will the fat cells in your butt, hips, arms, back, and cheeks. The last to budge will be the fat cells in your stomach, which is probably where you desperately desire to see the most change. Those abdominal fat cells were deemed the most important during pregnancy, and therefore, are crowned the most stubborn during the postpartum period. At twelve months postpartum, my abominable abdominal fat cells were still making their last stand.

#4 Crunch Those Abs

If you haven't started doing crunches yet, now is the time. Stomach crunches won't get rid of the fat on top of the muscles (only aerobic exercise will, and as I just informed you, it may take them a while to shrink), but they will tone the muscles, reshape them, and flatten them out, as long as you are doing them with the proper technique.

Here's the perfect crunch: lie down, knees bent, feet flat, hands behind your head, and elbows out. Tighten your abdominal muscles, press your lower back to the floor, and slowly lift your shoulders and upper back about three inches off the floor—hold steady for a second or two, then slowly come back down to the floor. Each crunch should take about seven or eight seconds. How long does it take for you to do a crunch now? You're probably doing one a second with quick, jerking movements. But quick crunches don't give you the same results, the contractions aren't held long enough to strengthen and condition the muscles. As you're timing your crunches with slow, purposeful contractions, also note your breathing. Do you inhale as you come up and exhale as you come down? Most people do, when in fact, we should be doing it the other way around—

exhaling up and inhaling down. When you exhale, you automatically pull in your stomach muscles and this helps them to lie flatter as they're toning and reshaping.

It's not necessarily how many crunches you do; it's how you do them. The same holds true if you are using Ab Rollers, Ab Masters, or ab machines. Do them right, do them three times a week, and do as many as you can before your muscles fatigue and the burning sensation gets to you. If you can do dozens upon dozens without feeling a thing, you're probably not doing them right. Because the written word can never replace one-on-one instruction, you may want to consult with a personal trainer to show you exactly how to tighten your tummy with crunches and how to vary them as your abdominal muscles strengthen.

#5 Lift Weights To Lose Weight

Over the last few years, exercise physiologists have come to a startling conclusion: Aerobic exercise is great for the heart, lungs, and fat cells, but it doesn't significantly increase muscle mass. You lost a few pounds of muscle during labor and delivery that needs to be regained, and the best way to regain lost muscle is to weight train.

To weight train and build muscle, you don't necessarily have to join a gym and use the weight machines with a hundred other people. The benefit of the machines is that they automatically get you into the right posture so that you don't have to worry about positioning. But you can also use hand and ankle weights, or, as they are often called, free weights. They're not free in cost (although they are inexpensive), but they do free you from cumbersome equipment. If weights aren't your bag, you can also strengthen and build muscle with large rubber bands, various yoga positions, Pilates exercises, calisthenics, or floor exercises—or you can simply work in your garden, carry in your groceries, or play horsey with your kids. Any movement that involves lifting weight—your own body weight, your child's weight, a hand weight, or even the weight of gardening tools, groceries, baby carriers, and strollers—is weight training and will build muscle.

I could go into specifics on how to lift weights, use rubber bands, or do yoga, Pilates, and floor exercises, but there are so many different options and techniques that it's best to find the right one for you. Take a class, visit a reputable gym, buy a good book that gives detailed guidance (Miriam Nelson's *Strong Women Stay Young* is excellent), watch an instructional video, or find a certified personal trainer who can tailor weight-training exercises to your body. Just make sure she or he has experience working with postpartum women, and make sure you get an okay from your doctor before you start weight training or any type of exercise program.

Once you find the right type of weight-training exercise for you, the overall goal is to do two thirty-minute sessions a week. Unlike aerobic exercise, these thirty-minute sessions do not have to be done all at once. You can break it up and spend 10 minutes in the morning before your baby gets up, 10 minutes during the day when she's napping, and 10 minutes at night while she's playing with Daddy. Or you can do your weight-training exercises during commercials or while watching a couple hours of TV. You need at least a day in between your two sessions to repair the muscle and get stronger. If Saturday and Sunday are your only options, do it early Saturday and late Sunday to have as much time as possible in between sessions.

To master postpartum fitness, you need both aerobics and weight training. Three hours of aerobic exercise a week will ensure fat release and one hour of weight training will guarantee muscle gain and a faster metabolism. Muscle is metabolically active tissue that burns calories all day long. More muscle and a faster metabolism mean a greater calorie-burning potential twenty-four hours a day.

Eat Write: The Pen Is Mightier Than the Fork

We all want to eat right, and the most successful way to get there is to "eat write"—to jot down everything you put into your body. And my definition of eating right differs from others you may have heard. It's not eating low-fat, low-cholesterol, low-sugar, and low-sodium foods; it's eating moderate portions of every food regardless of its fat, cholesterol, sugar, and sodium content. *It's eating moderate portions of every food, whether society has deemed it healthy or not.*

I've been an advocate of keeping food records for twenty years. I've strongly recommended it in my private practice and in my other books because I've always observed that those women who record what they ate lost a record amount of weight in record time. Up until recently, I never had a scientific explanation or documented research to back up my request—just anecdotal observations, which was never quite enough to win over the skeptics. Lisa was one of those skeptics. "Why should I keep food records? How much weight will I lose if I keep them? Where's the proof? And don't tell me it works because of the calories you burn during the writing process. I write all day long. I'm a copy editor, and it hasn't done me any good."

So, here's the proof: Researchers at the Center for Behavioral Research in Chicago found that those women who kept food records lost twice as much weight as those who didn't. And what about the proof specifically for postpartum women? I have that for you, too. Postpartum women were recently followed for six months, and those who kept food records (along with a regular walking program) lost 80 percent of their pregnancy weight. Those who didn't only lost 44 percent. Again, record-keeping resulted in almost twice the weight loss. So postpartum or not, *keeping food records will help keep your weight down.*

Even with this research, Lisa still wasn't 100 percent convinced, so I asked her to tell me what she ate yesterday, and she was stumped. "Yesterday . . . ummm . . . let me think . . . yesterday was what? Oh right, Tuesday. What happened Tuesday? Let's see, for breakfast I had cereal. No, that was this morning. Yesterday I had a doctor's appointment in the morning, so what did I eat? Oh, I remember. Nothing. I was too rushed getting ready and I forgot. Then, when I got home from the doctor's, I was starving, so I had something . . . but what was it? I know, a turkey sandwich. Then for dinner I had a baked potato, broccoli, and chicken."

Lisa had to use every available brain cell to remember what she ate twenty-four hours ago. Then as I asked for more specifics, she realized that her memory was worse than she thought, she had "forgotten the bad stuff." She remembered the turkey sandwich, but forgot the chips; recalled the broccoli and baked potato but neglected to mention the cheese sauce, butter, and sour cream; remembered the meals but got amnesia when it came to the snacks. Somewhere buried deep in our brains is a little voice that tells us if we don't remember it, it doesn't count and won't cause weight gain. Don't we wish! Everything counts. The sodas, juice, jelly beans, leftover sandwich crust from your son's plate, the snacks with your kids in the afternoon, the mouthfuls while you're preparing dinner, and the grazing while you're gazing at the TV.

Writing down what you eat improves your memory and makes an honest woman out of you. Not that you're a liar; just that you conveniently underestimate what you're eating by at least 20 percent, according to research at the University of Minnesota School of Public Health. And I don't necessarily blame you. No one wants to admit to eating the whole batch of cookie dough while the oven's preheating or an entire frozen cheesecake eaten directly from the freezer. What would your husband, mother, boss, therapist, doctor, or nutritionist think? They might outwardly condemn you, but internally, they'll be thinking about the last time they secretly did the same thing.

We are a nation of secretive eaters who won't admit our true eating habits for all the world to hear. We live in a society filled with eating morality and food fundamentalism, so why risk the possibility of judgment and condemnation? Butter is evil, so of course we don't eat it (wink, wink). Red meat is bad, and we'd never put a bad thing in our bodies (nudge, nudge). Sugar is white death, and we gave that up years ago (say no more). As a result, what we say we're eating and what we're really eating doesn't add up.

What We Say:	**What We Do:**
60 percent of us say that we are eating fewer sweets	We are eating nine pounds more sugar per year
70 percent of us say we are eating less fast food	The number of fast food customers has increased 6 percent
55 percent of us say that we are eating less butter and margarine	Consumption has stayed steady
56 percent of us say we are eating less ice cream	Consumption has stayed steady

Whether we consciously or unconsciously underestimate our eating, fudging about it is worse than eating fudge. Underestimating undermines your weight loss. If you don't admit to exactly what and how much you're eating, then you won't compensate by exercising a little more that day or eating a little less the next. That's why the pen is mightier than the fork. When you write it down, it's there in black and white, and you have no other option than to acknowledge *everything* you're eating.

So, get out your pen and start writing down what you're eating. You can use the food records that I've provided for you at the end of this chapter or you can order the *Postpartum Peace Plan Personal Eating Journal* on page 211 of the Additional Resources section. You can buy a fancy cloth journal or use stick-it pads. It doesn't matter. Just write—then analyze. I hope you're already eating smaller portions from the last chapter, but as you gaze at your day's intake, look for patterns. Do you eat too little food in the morning and too much at night? Are you still overeating at meals? Or do you feel stuffed mostly after eating snacks? Are you more likely to overindulge at home or in restaurants? Do you restrict certain foods, then overeat them? Or are you still overeating everything? In other words, what type of overeater are you?

- **The breakfast-skipper overeater.** One in four of us skip breakfast every day, and half of the rest eat breakfast only occasionally. Not a good weight-loss decision. Skipping breakfast causes us to eat more later in the day. It's the body's natural reaction to starvation—when we don't eat, our appetite center kicks into overdrive, sending us into an overeating frenzy, and we gain weight. Vanderbilt University showed that breakfast eaters lose twice as much weight as breakfast skippers. To stop overeating and start losing weight—start eating breakfast.

- **The variety-is-the-spice-of-life overeater.** Eating a variety of foods is healthy, but too much variety at any one meal may cause us to overeat because of something called sensory specific satiety—scientific jargon for the indisputable fact that the fifth bite of chocolate (or any other food) never tastes as good as the first. When you eat one food, you're satiated with a smaller amount because your taste buds get bored from the same taste. But when you eat many different foods at the same time, you need to eat enough of each food to satisfy your taste buds and reach a level of satiety. This explains why researchers at the University of Oxford found that when people were offered four different kinds of sandwiches, they ate 33 percent more than when they were just presented with one. These researchers also found that it's not just taste that determines satiation, but shape as well. When people were given three different shapes of pasta with tomato sauce, they ate 14 percent more than when they were given just one shape. The moral of this research: stay away from buffets, smorgasbords, pu-pu platters, and all-you-can-eat Italian dinners.

- **The kitchen-made-me-do-it overeater.** You're home, the kitchen's there, and you have to walk through it to get to the family room, bathroom, and laundry room—might as well check to see what's in the refrigerator while you're at it. Being at home with your baby means being at home with a ready supply of food. But don't blame the kitchen, you are responsible for opening up the refrigerator and inserting food into your mouth—and keeping records helps to make you more food-accountable.

- **The restaurant overeater.** This one probably hasn't applied to you over the last few months, but it may have before and definitely will in the very near future. Families with young children are the number one patrons of fast-food establishments, and parents of young children escape to restaurants as often as they can. And when we do, we eat more. Whether it's because we want to get our money's worth or because we eat more in social situations, the University of Memphis found that those women who eat out the most (five or more times a week) consumed an average of three hundred more calories and twenty more grams of fat a day. Restaurants don't have to ruin your weight loss goals—you can split a meal with your companion or take the rest home for tomorrow's lunch.

- **The fat-free overeater.** Fifty percent of us say that fat is our biggest dietary concern (only 8 percent say that it's calories), so food companies have enthusiastically responded with thousands of reduced-fat products, and we have eagerly filled our grocery carts with everything from nonfat cheese to fat-free cookies, and from reduced-fat Doritos to low-fat dog food. But neither we nor our canine friends are losing weight. How can that be? Because we're overeating fat-free foods, and fat-free does not mean calorie-free. As our fat intakes have come down in the last decade, our calorie intakes have actually gone up. Why stop at one cookie when they're fat-free? Why have a handful of chips when the whole bag contains no fat? Why wait until you get home from the grocery store to eat the fat-free crackers? Your baby's screaming in the backseat, your other two kids are fighting, you feel hopeless, and the crackers are right there beside you on the seat, ready to distract your senses from the nerve-racking noise.

"What about me?" asked Marilyn. "None of these eating types apply to me. I'm not an overeater at all. In fact, I'm probably not eating enough." Oh yes, I neglected to address the other pattern you may identify from your food records—undereating. Even though I've discussed ad nauseam the dangers of dieting and not eating enough during the postpartum months, Marilyn (and some of you) may have plugged your ears and skimmed over those sections. I took a look at Marilyn's food records and saw two foods repeated over and over again: yogurt and cucumbers. At first she tried to convince me that they were her favorite foods, then she finally admitted that she was on a yogurt and cucumber diet. "But it's supposed to make you lose ten pounds in ten days, so I just had to try it. And the convenient bonus is that it also doubles as a facial mask and takes ten years off of your face while it's taking ten pounds off your body." It most likely won't do either, but with the lack of carbohydrates, fat, vitamin C, beta-carotene, iron, zinc, and other nutrients, it may take ten years off your life.

Which brings me to the next valuable use of your food records: to assess your overall nutritional balance. Are you eating enough fruits and vegetables? You need at least five servings (1/2 cup portions) a day for good health, seven to eight if you're breastfeeding. Are you getting enough calcium? You need the equivalent of at least three eight-ounce glasses of milk (four to five if you are breastfeeding). Are you getting enough protein? You need at least two three-ounce servings a day (three if you're breastfeeding). Enough carbohydrates? Contrary to the slew of recent diet books, carbohydrates are not fattening unless you overeat them. You need at least six servings of carbohydrates a day (one slice of bread; one-half cup of rice, potato, pasta, or corn; and three-quarters of a cup of cereal) for energy, endurance, mood stability, and B vitamins. If you are still tentative about rice, pasta, potatoes, and bread—go global. The Chinese and Japanese eat rice, and they are lean. The French freely enjoy bread (as well as wine) and are famous for their lean bodies and low risk of heart disease. The Irish are potato lovers, and they don't have a weight problem. The Italians indulge in pasta, and it doesn't go straight to their hips. These countries all support the principle that *it's not what you eat—but how much you eat that counts.*

The world can also help you overcome your fat phobia. The Europeans eat real butter, real cheese, and extra virgin olive oil—they just don't overeat it. We, on the other hand, vacillate between eating too much fat and eating too little. Are you eating enough fat? Your body needs at least one high-fat food (and preferably two or three) every day to absorb the fat-soluble vitamins, keep your skin moist with natural oils, balance your hormones (estrogen is made from fat), and stabilize your moods. The University of Sheffield in England found that when women cut their fat intake about in half, their brains responded by making them moodier and more hostile. Has your family been complaining about your mood swings and hostile behavior? It may be due to your low-fat diet. Have you been complaining about your inability to lose weight? This could be due to your low-fat diet, too. When you don't eat enough fat, your body goes into a type of semistarvation state, dropping your metabolism and protecting your fat cells.

Keeping food records can do more than help you lose weight—they can also help you to balance your moods and maintain your health. As you begin keeping records, you may have some questions about how to do it. Here are some answers to commonly asked questions to help you eat write:

1. *Do I have to keep records right after I eat a meal or can I wait until the end of the day to write it all down?* You probably already know the answer to this question. If you wait until the end of the day,

you're bound to forget something. Postpartum memory loss can cause a raging case of eating amnesia, and you'll forget half of what you ate. But you can keep a mini tape recorder in your pocket and dictate your meals and snacks as you eat them, then write it all down at the end of the day when your kids are in bed and you have more time.

2. *What if I forget to bring my food journal with me to a restaurant or a friend's house?* Jessica kept forgetting to bring her journal with her, so right after she ate, she called her voice mail and left a detailed food message to herself.
3. *Are there any other options besides writing it down?* You can always type it in, but that means having your laptop with you everywhere you go. And with a baby, diaper bag, and rattles, there probably isn't any room left in the stroller.
4. *What if I miss a day or two?* No problem, just chalk it up to writer's block, and start again first thing the next morning. But don't let more than four days lapse, you'll find yourself overeating again.
5. *Do I have to keep food records for the rest of my life?* No, these next six months are the most important, but you may choose to continue because food records keep you focused and conscious of your eating.
6. *Why do some new mothers lose weight without keeping records?* Because some women are in tune with their bodies and fully aware of their eating habits without writing it down. But these women probably never (or seldom) dieted, and therefore, naturally have moderate eating habits that don't need to be changed.

Jessica had another question for me: "Why did my friend lose weight without doing *anything*? She didn't keep food records, she didn't exercise, she didn't decrease her portion sizes, and she lost every single ounce within three months without a trace of a stretch mark." The only answer I had was that her friend was simply not human—but an alien shape-changer who was sent to this planet to drive us earth girls crazy. She also probably never lost a lock of hair, leaked urine from her bladder, or was scared half to death by the sight of a spider vein. Why would she? She's not human.

Fat Isn't the Only Thing You Have to Outsmart: Hair Loss, Stretch Marks, Weak Bladders, and More

Over the next six months, you'll notice some other things happening to your body that at times will put weight loss at the bottom of your worry list. Your hair will start falling out, and you'll think you're going bald. Stretch marks will become more apparent as your belly completely deflates. Urine will sneak out of your bladder every time you cough, sneeze, jump, or laugh. Your period will start again, and PMS will attack in full force. Your energy will disappear, and you'll fantasize about running away to a spa and never coming back. And your decision about resuming outside employment may send you packing your bags for your biggest guilt trip ever. Welcome to motherhood. If fat cells were the only thing we had to outsmart, we could focus, take action, and shrink those little suckers with determination and efficiency. But these other postpartum anxiety producers get in the way, weigh heavy on our minds, and have to be outsmarted, too.

Lost Locks: Hair Today, Gone Tomorrow

Has it already started happening? Is your hair falling out in clumps? Is your tub filled with hair after a shower? Are you buying Drāno by the gallon? Don't call Rogaine yet—your hormones are wreaking havoc with your hair. Your hair will stop falling out (eventually) and will grow back (eventually). You'll have the tiny wisps of hair sticking straight up like I do right now to prove it.

During pregnancy, the high estrogen levels kept your hair permanently stuck in the growth cycle, so you didn't lose the one hundred hairs you were supposed to each day. That's why your hair felt thicker and more luxurious than normal, but that was just Mother Nature teasing us. Now, with estrogen levels at an all-time low, expect to lose as much as five hundred hairs a day. You're simply losing what you should have lost during pregnancy—all at once. You don't have a disease, you're not going bald—and getting stressed out about it may only lead to additional hair loss.

Until that glorious day when you see new hair growth (which may not be for another few months), eat nutritious foods, shampoo as infrequently as possible, use conditioner generously, let your hair dry naturally, postpone any perms or highlights, and get a really good hair cut.

Stretch Marks: Give Me an Eraser!

When your skin stretches 400 percent to accommodate your growing baby, it's bound to leave its mark. Think of a balloon: When you blow it up and then deflate it, it never quite goes back to its original compact size. Neither does your skin, and it leaves those deep, dark lines to forever remind you that you bore a child.

I can hear your protests all the way to Oakland, California. "But I know a woman who has a perfectly taut, stretch mark–free belly after having twins. I've seen photos of celebrities in lingerie looking like they never bore a child. I've stared at bikini-clad bodies at the beach, convincing myself that the woman swimming with the clan of kids can't possibly be the mother and must be the au pair." The truth is that some women simply don't get stretch marks. They are genetically blessed with highly elastic skin. They may also be twenty years old with youthful, more pliable skin. Both age and genetics determine whether or not a woman gets stretch marks.

For those of us who aren't twenty any more and were endowed with less stretchable skin, I'm sorry to say that there isn't much you can do to outsmart stretch marks. During pregnancy, you may have tried to prevent them with vitamin E oils and belly balms. Whether or not they helped, you'll never know—unless you do an experiment during your next pregnancy and apply nothing. Now that you have them, exercise won't erase the stretch marks, and your diet won't undo the damage.

But a dermatologist might. Laser surgery is becoming more popular for treating stretch marks, and some alpha-hydroxy products and prescription vitamin A creams have been found to lessen their appearance in some women. You can, however, take a nonsurgical, nonprescription approach to prevent them from getting worse—lose weight very slowly and never diet again for the rest of your life. Fast, frequent, and unhealthy weight fluctuations will enlarge your stretch marks and make them spread all over your belly, hips, buttocks, and thighs. Yet another reason to avoid drastic diets.

The Itsy, Bitsy Spider Veins

You have fifty-one thousand miles of arteries, veins, and capillaries running through your body, and the high estrogen levels during pregnancy dilated most of them and broke some of them. The result: spider veins and varicose veins. Spider veins are broken capillaries close to the skin that just couldn't take the pressure from increased blood flow. Varicose veins, a close cousin to spider veins, are larger, deeper, bulgier, and are caused by the pooling of blood. You may have one, the other, or both, in which case, you have sworn off any apparel that falls above the knee. Why do they invade our legs? Because the veins in our lower body have to work against gravity to get the blood back up to the heart. A hard enough job without the vein-weakening effects of estrogen.

What can you do about them? Elevating your feet and wearing support hose may have prevented them, but they won't do much good now. Or maybe you did elevate and support, but got them anyway. Dismal news, but here's something that will make you happy:

Your varicose veins may diminish or even disappear on their own. Without the pressure of your uterus on your leg veins, there's a good chance that they may start to pump the pooled blood back up to your heart, and you'll wake up one morning pleasantly surprised. Now for some more dismal news: spider veins are here to stay—unless you decide to go the cosmetic surgery route with lasers or sclerotherapy, a technique that collapses the spider vein and is effective in 90 percent of the cases.

Constipation: This Too Shall Pass

Passing your first stool after delivery was tantamount to passing a kidney stone. And since that painful day, you may have had a problem with constipation. Pregnancy slowed down the smooth muscle contractions of your colon, and it may take them awhile to get back up to speed. Then, some of you also have hemorrhoids that formed during pregnancy and/or during the bearing down and pushing hours of delivery. No matter how painful or uncomfortable it may be to have a bowel movement—don't suppress the urge. The longer the stool sits in the colon, the more water is drawn from it, the harder it gets, and the harder it becomes for you to have a bowel movement.

To shake things up a bit and keep it moving:

- **Eat plenty of fiber.** High-fiber cereals, whole-grain breads, and fresh fruits and vegetables contain roughage that isn't digested or absorbed, so it provides bulk to your stool. It also provides fullness to your stomach, satisfying you for a longer time and helping you lose weight. Bulking agents like Metamucil and Fiberall contain large amounts of fiber, but they are not food, so you're not getting the other nutrients along with it.

- **Drink plenty of water.** Without water, a high-fiber diet can constipate you even more. Your stool needs water to stay moist, soft, and in transit.

- **Keep moving.** Exercise relaxes the mind, shakes up the colon, and makes your bowels more cooperative.

- **Use laxatives sparingly.** If you take them too often, your colon may become dependent on them, versus working to get its smooth muscles contracting again.

If you're not constipated, you may have another, more embarrassing bowel problem: Fecal incontinence. You can't hold it back, and it leaks out all on its own. A vaginal delivery stretches out the muscles between your vagina and anus so much that the anal sphincter might not be working as it should. Six percent of postpartum women report a problem with fecal incontinence—that's probably more than you thought, but it's not something women bring up in dinner conversation. What can you do about leaky stools? Kegel exercises help to strengthen the pelvic floor muscles and are the solution to both types of incontinence: fecal and urinary.

What's the Matter with My Bladder?

One in six new mothers still experience some degree of urinary incontinence months after birth, and if you're one of them, it most likely started during your pregnancy when the weight of your uterus weakened the ligaments of your bladder—and continues now because labor and delivery stretched the connective tissue that supports your bladder and urethra. To cope with a "weak bladder," some women restrict their fluids, but that dehydrates the body and increases the risk of urinary tract infections and constipation. Some women won't exercise for fear of leakage, but that prevents you from burning fat. Others won't leave the house even if they have Depends, but that prevents you from living.

Almost all women find relief with Kegel exercises. The *Journal of the American Medical Association* recently reported on a study that showed an 81 percent improvement in urinary incontinence with Kegel exercises. Not just a dozen pelvic floor tightening exercises a day, but a hundred or more (see chapter 4 for a review of the technique if you didn't do them immediately after delivery as suggested). If you want to be out of diapers before your baby is—do your Kegels. They really help.

It's Back: PMS Attacks!

After fifteen glorious, PMS-free months, 80 percent of you will start your period during this time. And the first one could be a doozy—sending your family running for cover and you running to Godiva for a chocolate binge. So be on the lookout for that out-of-sorts, out-of-control, out-of-your-mind state of mind that is a telltale sign. When stress is high, patience is low, and moods are everywhere across the board, you may be about to start your first period. If your partner asks, "Do you have PMS or something?" don't deny it with an explosion of expletives. He may know your PMS moods better than you; trust his awarenesses. After all, we seldom have PMS mood swings when we're alone, now do we?

Give your PMS some TLC:

- **Take calcium supplements.** The *American Journal of Obstetrics and Gynecology* recently reported that twelve hundred mg of calcium significantly reduced fourteen signs and symptoms of PMS.

- **Indulge in chocolate.** It helps; I kid you not. It's been found to increase endorphins and serotonin in our brains and mimic the feeling of falling in love (with the chocolate, not your spouse). But all you need is half an ounce for a calmer, tamer PMS—the equivalent of a third of a candy bar or two Hershey's Kisses.

- **Eat small, frequent meals.** PMS attacks are more likely to occur when our blood-sugar level is low. Little meals eaten throughout the day keep blood-sugar levels high and PMS low.

The New Mom Energy Crisis

You've recovered from labor, you're getting at least a little more sleep each night, and you're exercising and eating healthy—so why do you feel even more tired than you did a couple of months ago? Because you've got the most demanding job in the universe. You're working twenty-four hours a day, seven days a week. You're expending massive amounts of energy breastfeeding your baby, taking care of your baby, taking care of your other kids, taking care of the house, taking care of the meals, taking care of the car, taking care of the dog, and now others are asking you to take care of them. Family is starting to call asking for favors, friends are starting to call asking for help, volunteer organizations are starting to call asking for your skills, and your office is starting to call asking for your advice. After all, you're on maternity leave, so you have the time. Right? Wrong. Motherhood is the hardest job I've ever had, making both time and energy precious commodities.

Without long-term solutions to your energy crisis, you'll be fatigued for weeks, months, and maybe years to come. Another of my books, *Outsmarting Female Fatigue,* reveals natural, lasting strategies to add energy to each day—but let me highlight a few of the fatigue-fighting keys that have been most helpful to my postpartum clients.

- **Let the sunshine in.** Get natural light every day, especially in the morning. It boosts brain serotonin and gives you increased energy all day long. How about walking with your baby in the morning? You'll both start the day with a revitalized outlook.

- **Start saying "no" to others demanding your energy.** It's too precious, and you need every single bit of it for you and your baby. You might as well start feeling comfortable with the word "no" now. You'll be hearing a lot of it soon; it was my Tyler's first word and continues to be his favorite.

- **Sip water throughout the day.** Dehydration is the number one cause of fatigue, and postpartum women are dehydrated. You lost fluid through blood loss, night sweats, and breastmilk production. And if you're anything like the typical American woman, you're only drinking two glasses of water a day, but need six to eight.

- **Take deep belly breaths.** It increases oxygen circulation in your blood, and your cells need oxygen to make energy. Most of us are shallow breathers; we breathe through our chests and not through our bellies. Watch your baby breathe, his or her whole body expands on the inhale. Let your baby teach you something—how to breathe.

If you don't deal with your fatigue, you won't have the energy to exercise, play with your baby, get together with your friends, have sex with your partner, or go back to work—if you've come to that decision yet.

Guilt Trips: Should I Stay or Should I Go?

Guilt may be nothing new to you. You felt guilty before you got pregnant (about the cookies you ate, the check you bounced, the car you scratched, the birthday you missed), and you felt guilty during your pregnancy (the medication you took before you knew, and the wine and coffee you drank after you knew). Now, you feel guilty for a multitude of things: your baby's first cold, not being able to breastfeed, being perfectly able to breastfeed but choosing not to, not exercising enough, exercising too much, and spending too much time away from your baby—to mention just a few. But according to a number of surveys, our biggest guilt producer is "the decision" about staying at home or going back to work.

Either way you decide can produce guilt. If you go back to work, you may feel guilty that you're not home spending enough time with your baby. If you stay at home, you may feel guilty that you're not advancing your career, contributing income to the family, or spending enough *quality time* with your baby and other children. Whatever your decision, feeling guilty about it only makes you less effective as a mother and a worker. Find some realistic solutions instead. Maybe you can negotiate a longer maternity leave or a three- or four-day work week. Perhaps you can find a day-care facility close to work. Or maybe you can find a new job that offers on-site day care. You may not be able to control your decision about going back to work, but you *can* control your work environment and attitude.

It may give you peace of mind to know that research shows children of working mothers are just as secure, emotionally adjusted, and intellectually developed as those of stay-at-home moms. If you still have tears in your eyes at the thought of leaving your baby, maybe this will help: Research has also shown that working mothers lose more weight than stay-at-home mothers. No one knows exactly why, but a number of studies have shown the same results. It may be that working mothers put more pressure on themselves to lose the weight for fear that their coworkers will judge them. Or it may be that working mothers have fewer opportunities to eat with no kitchen right around the corner.

Instead of wasting time and energy feeling guilty about anything—direct that attention back to your baby and your body. Your baby needs your full attention and care, and your body needs your focus to lose weight. So tilt the guilt and treasure the pleasure of being a mother who loves her baby—and being a woman who is successfully outsmarting her fat cells.

WHAT'S YOUR POSTPARTUM PEACE PLAN FOR THE NEXT SIX MONTHS?

These six months are your window of opportunity to really outsmart postpartum fat; this is when aerobic exercise will burn fat, and moderate eating will shrink fat cells. So, what's your plan? What specific changes will you make? Check all that make sense for your new lifestyle, and all that you will work on for the next 180 days.

What Will You Do to Pamper Yourself?

____ I will think positively about my body and its ability to lose weight.

____ I will throw my body a surprise party with a bubble bath, facial mask, scented lotion, and relaxing music.

____ I will take care of my hair by using gentle shampoo, conditioner, and letting it air dry.

____ I will energize my tired body with sunshine, laughter, water, and deep belly breaths.

____ I will take care of my bowels by eating more fiber, drinking more water, and exercising.

What Will You Do to Eat With a Regular Meal Schedule?

____ I will "eat write" by keeping food records and honestly recording my eating.

____ I will use my food records to identify patterns of overeating and practice realistic solutions.

____ I will use my food records to assess the nutritional balance of my diet—making sure that I'm eating enough fruits and vegetables, dairy products, protein foods, and grains.

____ I will include some fat in my diet to balance my mood, produce estrogen, prevent the starvation response, and help me lose weight.

____ I will record what I eat after every meal and snack, and if I don't have my records with me or I don't have the time, I'll write it down on a napkin, dictate it into a tape recorder, or call it in to my voice mail.

What Will You Do to Actively Move Your Body?

____ I will exercise aerobically, slowly building up to forty-five minutes three to five times a week.

____ I will somehow, some way find the time to exercise: I'll walk with my baby, hire a babysitter, trade babysitting time with a friend, work out at a gym that offers child care, or wait until my partner gets home from work.

____ I will slow down my pace and exercise at a moderate intensity.

____ I will monitor my rate of breathing with the talk test—making sure that I can complete short sentences before needing to take a breath.

____ I will practice the proper technique for doing crunches by breathing in on the lift and taking seven to eight seconds with slow, purposeful movements.

____ I will lift weights, use rubberbands, or take a strength-training class two days a week to rebuild my muscle mass and boost my metabolism.

____ I will consult a personal trainer for one-on-one instruction with weight lifting and crunches if I need to.

What Will You Do to Calm Your Stress?

____ I will have the patience to lose weight slowly over these next six months.

____ I will realize that some hair loss is normal, and my hair will grow back.

____ I will realize that stretch marks, varicose veins, and spider veins are normal and a souvenir of pregnancy.

____ I will be aware of the possibility of a first PMS attack and will help calm its intensity with calcium supplements, chocolate, and small, frequent meals.

____ I will not waste time and energy feeling guilty about *anything*.

What Will You Do to Embrace Your New Body?

___ I will imagine how my life would change if I woke up tomorrow morning liking my body.

___ I will stand straight and tall and walk with confidence.

___ I will talk back to that inner critical voice that tells me I'm overweight and worthless.

___ I will initiate sex to boost my self-esteem.

___ I will give myself body compliments, give others compliments, and accept compliments from others.

___ I will go to an art museum to realize that my voluptuous body is a work of art.

___ I will become an advocate for body acceptance by joining an organization, writing letters to fashion magazines, buying *Mode* magazine, and/or talking about body image with my friends and daughters.

___ I will find five things I like about my body and acknowledge them every day.

Food Record

These records have nothing to do with counting calories or grams of fat, and they will not be looked at by anyone but you. So, be honest and use them to identify patterns and areas to focus on. Write with longhand or shorthand, a fancy calligraphy pen or a #2 pencil from your child's backpack. All that matters is that you "eat write" every day. Here is an example and a blank record for you to use. You can also design your own or order the *Postpartum Peace Plan Personal Eating Journal* (see Additional Resources).

Meal/ Snack	Time of Day	Were You Hungry Before Eating?	What Did You Eat	How Did You Feel After Eating?
breakfast	6:45 am	yes	1 c cereal	satisfied
			1 c milk	and
			1/2 c orange juice	comfortable
snack	9:30 am	a little	1 c yogurt	good
			1 banana	refreshed
			glass of water	
lunch	12:15 pm	yes	1/2 sandwich	not full!
			some baby carrots	
			a few chips	the chips
			iced tea	tasted great
snack	4:00 pm	very!	other 1/2 sandwich	energized
			1 chocolate cookie	and
			glass of milk	productive
dinner	7:15 pm	yes	1 chicken breast	satisfied
			1/2 c rice	and a little
			1 c spinach	tired
			water	

Comments I visualized portions and ate smaller more frequent meals. I gave my body fruits, vegetables, protein, and carbohydrate and even some fat, chips, and chocolate. It was a great day!

FOOD RECORD

MEAL/ SNACK	TIME OF DAY	WERE YOU HUNGRY BEFORE EATING?	WHAT DID YOU EAT?	HOW DID YOU FEEL AFTER EATING?

COMMENTS

Chapter Seven

The Next Six Years: The Birth of a New, Happy, Healthy You

It is my sincere hope that as you enter this next phase of your postpartum life, you have a greater acceptance and appreciation of your miraculous female body, that you believe in your ability to outsmart your postbaby fat cells, and that you've experienced enough positive changes in your body to know that the Postpartum Peace Plan is working for you.

I don't expect that many of you have reached your prepregnancy weight. In fact, research suggests that most of you haven't; only one third of women are within five pounds of their prepregnancy weight at nine months. So, if you're not, it's perfectly acceptable. Your body just started burning fat six months ago, your baby probably just started sleeping through the night (if you're lucky), and your life has just started having some semblance of a routine. But here's what I do expect: that you have lost some of the weight, that your fat cells are noticeably smaller, that your muscles are more toned, and that you are fitting into most (or at least some) of your prepregnancy clothes. In other words, I expect that your body is at least moving in the right direction.

If you feel that your body is not moving much of anywhere, it's time to take a good, hard look at your commitment to the eating and exercise strategies of the Postpartum Peace Plan.

- **Have you *really* been working on body acceptance?** Because you won't lose weight and keep it off until you do.
- **Have you *really* been exercising aerobically for forty-five minutes, three to five times a week?** Because your fat cells won't shrink until you do.
- **Have you *really* been doing crunches?** Because your stomach muscles won't strengthen, tighten, and flatten until you do.
- **Have you *really* been weight training?** Because you won't regain your shape, tone your muscles, and boost your metabolism until you do.
- **Have you *really* been eating moderate portions?** Because your fat cells won't stop growing until you do.
- **Have you *really* been keeping food records?** Because you can't successfully monitor and change your eating habits until you do.

When I posed these questions to Nancy, who was convinced that the Postpartum Peace Plan wasn't working for her, she thought for a moment and responded, "The easy answer would be to tell you 'yes,' but in all honesty, I'm not really doing these things. I try, but with a baby, toddler, preschooler, and second grader, my life is one big roller coaster. I'm able to keep food records and maintain my exercise program for a couple of weeks, then I get overwhelmed trying to juggle everything between home and work—and freefall back down to where I started six months ago. I really want to slim down, but I guess I haven't been consistent enough. Is that why I haven't lost much weight?"

That's precisely why Nancy hadn't lost the weight, and that's why all of you who are discouraged haven't lost the weight, too. Whether this is your first child or fourth, whether you are juggling car pools or company politics (or both), whether you are married with a traveling spouse or single and going it all on your own—consistency will be a constant challenge. There will always be a sick child, a doctor's appointment, a flat tire, a broken appliance, a meeting, a school science project, or a soccer game that will understandably get in the way.

But you have to be consistent to outsmart those postpartum pounds. You can't eat moderately half the time, and overeat the other half. You can't exercise for forty-five minutes on some days, and only fifteen minutes on others. You can't lift weights one week, and skip the next. Your fat cells won't quite believe that you're trying to outsmart them. Sometimes you're teaching them how to release fat, and other times you're encouraging them to store. Eventually they'll get fed up, complaining that you can't make up your mind what you want them to do, and they'll not do anything—except stay fat and happy.

The fact is: Most of us aren't quite consistent enough. Even though 50 percent of us are trying to lose weight at any given moment, only 20 percent of us are consistent enough with our eating and exercise program to make it happen. If you're one of the 80 percent who aren't consistent enough, then it's time to make the Postpartum Peace Plan an integral part of your life. If this is your first child, it may be a bit easier now than six months ago—your baby isn't a newborn anymore, your support system is in place, and although time is still limited, you at least have a schedule that you can use to figure out how to fit in exercise. If this is your second, third, or fourth child, not much of anything will come easy, so you'll have to put a bit more creativity into making regular exercise and moderate eating a priority in your life. For some ideas and individualized support, you may want to consult with a registered dietitian for private counseling or a licensed therapist for help with body acceptance and behavioral change. At minimum, I recommend going back to the last chapter and starting the fat-burning part of the Postpartum Peace Plan again with a renewed commitment to be as consistent as you possibly can. *You won't outsmart your fat cells until you do.*

"But I have been consistent!" exclaimed Jenny, another client. "I answered 'yes' to all those questions. I've been faithfully exercising for forty-five minutes three times a week, lifting weights and doing crunches, and writing down what I eat—and I'm still struggling with eight more pounds to lose! If my fat cells don't shrink soon, I'm going to have to call a shrink. I can't live the rest of my life eight pounds heavier." If you've been consistent but still feel like you're struggling with the last few pounds, let me inform you that you're not struggling: You're normal. Those last few pounds (whether they be five, eight, or ten) are so infamously stubborn that the medical profession has coined them the "retained weight of pregnancy," but that doesn't necessarily mean that you're destined to retain them forever.

It's Not over Yet: Outsmarting the Last Few Pounds

Just when you thought you had your fat cells figured out with the Postpartum Peace Plan, they throw you a curve ball by refusing to shrink all the way down. With your peaceful, nondieting efforts, they have shrunk significantly, but all of a sudden, they are being very possessive about their last few pounds of pregnancy fat. You can't blame them. Pregnancy was the most fun they ever had; they got to store for nine months straight and fulfill their purpose in life. Now, they want to keep some pregnancy fat as a souvenir of their fat-storing heyday. And even more important, they want to hold on to some precious storage to give you a head start for your next pregnancy, or depending on your age, a jump on perimenopause (more on this later in this chapter). They'll need to grow anyway during these times, so they think that they're actually doing you a favor by keeping you a few pounds heavier.

So much for favors—this is one you could probably do without. Since you can't deprogram your fat cells or force out that stubborn leftover fat, you have to slowly encourage them to release their prized souvenir. It may take another three to six months to peacefully outsmart those last few pounds, but that's a timeline you have to accept and live with.

Jenny decided that she couldn't live with it. Her twenty-year high school reunion was a month away, and her mission was to blast away the last eight pounds to show all her classmates how three pregnancies and twenty years hadn't changed her body a bit. So, without informing me, she doubled her exercise program, thinking that twice the time would burn twice the fat. After three weeks of walking six days a week for two hours each day, she frantically called me up. "Help! I've gained two pounds. How can this be? I'm exercising so much I should be burning fat like an incinerator, but instead I've started storing fat again."

Exercise does outsmart your female fat cells, but with too much exercise, your fat cells end up outsmarting you. They have a built-in defense system when exercise starts to threaten their livelihood. If you exercise for much longer than an hour, that defense mechanism kicks in, and they start biting their nails with nervous tension. "Oh no. I've been releasing fat for the last thirty minutes, and she looks like she has no intention of stopping any time soon. But I can't release any more; she needs me. What if she gets pregnant tonight and a famine hits tomorrow? I better play it on the safe side by turning off fat burning for a while and starting to store again. I hope she eats something good for dinner tonight."

When I explained this overexercise–weight gain response to Jenny, she decided to go back to her original forty-five-minute fat-burning exercise program, but it was three days before her reunion, and as a result of overexercising, she now had ten pounds to lose. Discouraged and exasperated, she sheepishly asked about *The Celebrity Ten Pounds in Ten Hours Miracle Diet*. "Can I try that? I've seen the advertisements everywhere; it promises a ten pound loss in ten hours—and I'm desperate." Diets just love desperate women, and this one has all of the "can't resist" words. "Celebrity" is a sure sell—we're eager to try anything remotely related to the stars. "Lose ten pounds in ten hours" sounds just about right for our impatient natures—we'd like it gone yesterday, but later today would be acceptable and just in time for Jenny's reunion this weekend. "Miracle diet"—we've been searching for one most of our adult lives, and this could be it.

But Jenny's common sense told her it wasn't. The only thing she'd lose in ten hours would be her $39.95 investment. So, she went to the reunion ten pounds heavier and was pleasantly surprised to find that she was one of the fittest females there, and then even more pleased when half the class greeted her with compliments. Before Jenny left my office she asked, "I promise I won't do anything crazy like overexercise or try a liquid diet, but is there anything I can do to speed up the fat-burning process?"

The two most important things you can do to keep losing weight are (1) having the patience to wait out the next few months, and (2) being consistent with your exercise and eating. But there are four other strategies that may teach your fat cells some new tricks by subtly encouraging them to release more fat.

1. **Add another day of exercise.** If you are doing three days a week, add a fourth. If you're doing four days a week, add a fifth. But there is no need to do six or seven days a week; at five you reach a fat-burning plateau—and rest is an important component of fitness. You probably don't have time to exercise every day, anyway. Unless you have a full-time nanny, cook, and house cleaner, you barely have the time to fit three days into your busy schedule. If it is simply not humanly possible to add another day of exercise, skip this strategy and focus on one of the others.

2. **Add another five, ten, or fifteen minutes to your forty-five minute aerobic exercise sessions.** You may not be able to add a

day, but can you add five, ten, or fifteen minutes? Most of my clients say that's feasible, and just about all of them feel a fat-burning boost when they do. Since every minute after thirty minutes is a fat-burning minute, you'll see more change in your body exercising three times a week for sixty minutes than if you exercised four times a week for forty-five minutes—because you'll have more total fat-burning time. For example, if you walked an extra fifteen minutes three days a week, making it a full hour of aerobic exercise per session and ninety fat-burning minutes for the week, you could lose an extra four pounds of fat over the next six months.

3. **Change your activity.** Your fat cells get used to the same activity over and over again, but when you introduce something new, they are brought to attention. Try bike riding, stair climbing, a kick-boxing class, or even rollerblading. Your fat cells won't know what hit them. "Hey, those aren't sneakers she's putting on. Those things have wheels on them. What on earth is she going to do with wheels?" And when you take off down the street, it's a completely different movement that your fat cells aren't used to. They have no idea how much fat they'll need to release to fuel your rollerblading movements—so they release as much as they can, as quickly as they can.

4. **Vary your activity.** Having one or two activities that you rotate keeps your fat cells at a higher level of release because they never get used to one particular movement. You can walk on one exercise day, and go to an aerobics class the next. Or you can walk with your baby every exercise day, but just switch from jogger to backpack to jogger again. The goal is to keep your fat cells guessing.

Please keep in mind that you don't have to change anything about your exercise program to continue to outsmart your postpartum fat cells. If you don't have the time or the desire to increase the duration, frequency, or number of different activities—simply keep exercising three times a week for forty-five minutes. Then take a few deep breaths to summon the patience to stick with it for another three to six months. And while you're exercising and patiently waiting, acknowledge how far you've come and how much your fat cells have responded to your efforts.

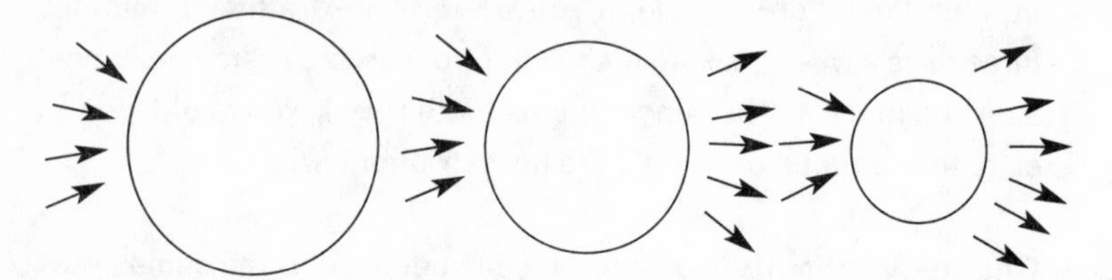

Where You Were Right After Birth | Where You Are Now | Where You Will Be Soon

You are making progress; your fat cells are storing less fat and releasing more, but please take another couple of deep breaths. Because when it's all said and done and your weight loss has stopped for good, you may find that your body is not exactly where you thought it would be. You may still be carrying an extra couple of pounds, you may still have a tough time buttoning some of your pants, and you may still have to take a refresher course in body acceptance. *Pregnancy is a life-altering, body-changing miracle. How could your body possibly remain unchanged after the miracle of birth?*

It's the Same Body, Only Different

In another few months, your fat loss will stop and your body weight will stabilize. It's impossible to predict exactly where your weight will stabilize, but I can tell you that the majority of women find that their new postpartum weight feels a little heavier, and their new postpartum body feels slightly different. It still accomplishes the same things for you as it did in your prepregnancy days—it still moves you to where you need to go, it still pumps blood and nutrients to your cells, it still breathes in oxygen to keep you alive, and it still sleeps to replenish itself. But now, with your baby forever on your mind, your body does these basic functions with a different purpose. When it moves, it responds to your baby's distress calls, traveling at the speed of light to take you where you need to go. When it pumps blood, it has the memory of transporting nutrients to your baby's developing cells and milk to your baby's mouth. When it breathes, it takes in the smell of your baby to keep you smiling and happy. When it sleeps, it reminisces about your baby's delivery and dreams of your baby's future. And when it does all these beautiful things, it does them with a few extra pounds, slightly wider hips, a little looser skin, a little more cellulite, and a few stretch marks and varicose veins.

Pregnancy has caused a physical, emotional, and spiritual transformation that will stay with you forever—and keep you healthier forever. Women who have children live longer, with a lower risk of physical and mental illness than women who don't have children. So, yes, pregnancy changed you, but it changed you for the better. And, yes, your body is different now, but it is healthier, too.

- **Your breasts are different and healthier.** After pregnancy and breastfeeding, it's doubtful your breasts will be as pert, firm, or big as they were before. As a client once said, "After having boobs big enough to have their own area code, I can now barely find them even with directory assistance." They may be smaller, but they're healthier. Pregnancy and breastfeeding lowered your risk of breast cancer by making the tissue less susceptible to possible cancer-causing substances.

- **Your ovaries are different and healthier.** Some women become more fertile after having a first child, with the ovaries releasing eggs each month with precision. But in addition to increased fertility, pregnancy also lowered your risk of ovarian cancer.

- **Your bones are different and healthier.** As long as you consumed enough calcium during pregnancy, your bone density increased. Carrying around a seven-pound fetus and another thirty pounds of extra tissue and fluids forced your bones to get stronger and reduced your risk of osteoporosis.

- **Your feet are different and healthier.** They are a half-size bigger than before, and although I couldn't find any physical health benefit to larger feet, there is a possible mental health benefit—you get to buy all new shoes in the latest styles.

- **Your hips are different and healthier.** Some women's hips never quite go back into place after expanding half a foot during labor; mine didn't. The health benefit of wider hips is that your next baby should be delivered with greater ease.

- **Your brain is different and healthier.** For starters, it's happier. Assuming that any baby blues or postpartum depression is a distant memory, mothers report more joy, balance, and satisfaction—and are 30 percent less likely than women without children to become clinically depressed. As a result of pregnancy, your brain also has a quicker reaction time and is better equipped to handle multiple tasks. How else could you feed your baby, prepare dinner, talk on the phone to your office, and catch a falling glass of milk in midair before it hits the floor—all at the same time?

- **Your body weight is different and healthier.** Carrying a few extra pounds doesn't kill you; in fact, the opposite may be true. It may help you live longer. A number of studies have investigated the lower death rates of normal weight and moderately overweight people, but they have received little or no media attention in this

> thin-obsessed country. These studies have been done at reputable institutions across the nation (such as Stanford, Cornell, and the National Institute of Aging) on huge numbers of people (300,000 to 600,000 subjects) and have found that the extreme underweight and overweight have higher mortality rates, but everyone in between (including those who retain a few pounds from pregnancy) can live long, healthy lives.

Pregnancy affected every organ, every cell, every body part—every part of your life. But that was the whole point, wasn't it?

From Here to Maternity: Preparing for Your Next Pregnancy

"Are you going to have another one?" I can't begin to count the number of times I've been asked that question, and if I'm asked once more, I'm tempted to say that I'm having five more. The truth is, I don't know. I'm forty-one years old and happy with one child—at least for right now. If you, too, are grappling with the decision, you can always take the late (and greatly missed) Erma Bombeck's advice: never have more children than you have car windows. So, I'm leaning toward a two-seater convertible. If you're thinking about a minivan, all I can say is—better you than me.

Contemplating another child isn't the only decision you have to make. Your next hurdle is to decide when to get pregnant again. Maybe that decision will be made for you with a "little mistake," but since the advent of birth control, most of you are in the driver's seat. Do you wait two years like many of the books recommend to give your body plenty of time to fully recover? Do you listen to your friend who says do it right now and get it over with; your kids will be able to play together and keep themselves occupied? Or do you listen to your sister who says three years is the charm because you'll never have two in diapers at the same time? Don't listen to anyone but your own inner voice. There is no best time. Whenever you feel ready is the right time for you.

The right time for Alice was when she finished outsmarting her postpartum fat cells. She wanted to lose the weight and get in shape before her fat cells exploded again with another pregnancy. Not a bad plan. But it wouldn't be the end of the world if her plan didn't go according to plan and she got pregnant this week. Women with close pregnancies have as good a weight-loss prognosis as women who wait. They just have to outsmart their combined pregnancy weight gains at the same time—after their second baby is born.

If you've decided on another baby, forget about weight loss for right now. You can finish outsmarting your current postpartum fat cells after delivering your next child. Your primary goal is to have a healthy, thriving baby and be a healthy, vibrant mother. And it starts the minute you give in to that maternal desire to hold another newborn in your arms. It takes about four months to build up your nutritional status to a level that will benefit your pregnant body and developing baby. So pull out your prenatal vitamins (and make sure they have folic acid to prevent neural tube defects), and continue eating well and taking care of yourself.

Having already gone through at least one pregnancy, I'm assuming you know the basics of prenatal nutrition. Instead, I want to give you some information that you may not be familiar with. We'll call it *Your Ten Tips for Outsmarting a Difficult (and Unhealthy) Pregnancy,* and as you'll notice, these tips have many similarities to the Postpartum Peace Plan. So, no need to stop your eating and exercise program—just enhance them for your pregnancy needs.

1. **Don't restrict.** This one comes as no surprise; I'm an antidieting nutritionist who has lashed out against restriction a number of times already. But during pregnancy, it's absolutely essential that you don't deprive your growing baby of calories and nutrients. Not only is there an increased risk of premature birth, low birth weight, and fetal mortality, but there is also a chance that restriction may

cause problems for your child later on in life: learning difficulties, increased risk of heart disease, and obesity. If you try to prevent weight gain for you, you may be causing it for your child in adulthood. In a landmark study of the Dutch famine back in the 1940s, pregnant women were rationed only one thousand calories a day. They delivered smaller babies, but when those babies were studied fifty years later, they had become overweight adults. Why? It's thought that early starvation triggers an increase in fat-cell numbers—and the more fat cells you're born with, the more likely you'll struggle with weight.

2. **Don't use pregnancy as an excuse to overeat.** For the first trimester, your baby's growth is slow, and its need for calories minimal (it's only the size of a green bean). Your hunger should increase some, but not enough to be part owner of Ben & Jerry's Ice Cream. In fact, the addition of one glass of milk a day satisfies your increased caloric needs. During the second and third trimesters, your body needs more calories, but not nearly as much as you think. An extra two glasses of milk or a turkey and cheese sandwich is all it takes to supply the additional three hundred calories a day your baby requires for growth. All in all, it takes about sixty thousand calories to nourish a developing baby. That sounds like a lot, but it's spread over about 270 days. For comparison, if you eat a banana split every day of your pregnancy, your total intake will exceed 126,000 calories—half of which will be directed to your baby. The other half will be gobbled up by your fat cells.

3. **Gain whatever weight is appropriate for you.** Although the Institute of Medicine recommends a twenty-five- to thirty-five-pound weight gain, that may be too little, too much, or just right for you. Larger women usually need to gain less weight, and petite women usually need to gain more. Just ask my sister who's 4'11" and weighed eighty-eight pounds before she got pregnant. During her first pregnancy, she started showing at sixteen weeks and

gained forty-five pounds. During her second pregnancy, she popped at ten weeks, was wearing a full maternity wardrobe at fourteen weeks, and gained forty-four pounds. During her third pregnancy, she pulled out her maternity clothes as soon as her at-home test turned pink and gained forty-six pounds (basically the same in all three pregnancies, showing that our bodies are programmed to gain the weight they need to). Thankfully, she had the presence of mind to stop after three, and in case you were wondering, she has lost virtually all her pregnancy weight. But then again, look who she has for a sister.

4. **Trust your food cravings.** The most amazing food craving research was done in Thailand, where pregnant women were observed eating rotting wood. Not just one or two, but all the pregnant women in the village. The researchers were baffled until they discovered that the bacteria decomposing the wood were producing the exact B vitamins that were lacking in the women's diets. Isn't that amazing? During no other time in your life will your body communicate with you more strongly. And as this research shows, your body communicates via food cravings for specific reasons. What could possibly be the reason for ice cream? Your body needs the combination of calcium, fat, sugar, protein, and calories. Pickles? Sodium. Sardines? Salt, protein, zinc, and calcium. Chocolate? Brain euphoria. The magnesium, sugar, fat, and phenylethylamine (a chemical that mimics the feeling of falling in love) all boost positive brain chemicals. But don't fool yourself. Pregnancy food cravings don't surface the night of conception; it takes about eight weeks for pregnancy hormones to influence your appetite center and trigger food cravings.

5. **Trust your food aversions.** Do you have a bionic pregnancy nose? The smell, more than the taste, of food can turn you off and sometimes make you run for the nearest bathroom. The three top pregnancy food aversions are coffee, alcohol, and raw fish—all

something that our bodies can live without, and probably should live without during pregnancy. Too much caffeine isn't healthy for you or your baby, alcohol may interfere with your baby's brain development, and raw foods may carry listeria bacteria, which can cause a dangerous food-borne illness. Cook meats, fish, and poultry well, wash raw fruits and vegetables, and scrub hands, knives, and cutting boards after handling any raw foods.

6. **Keep exercising.** If you didn't exercise before and during your last pregnancy, you'll be pleasantly surprised at the outcome this time. Not only will you develop fewer varicose veins and have a lower risk of gestational diabetes and prenatal hypertension, you'll also most likely have a shorter, less-complicated labor. A number of studies have found that women who exercise aerobically at least three times a week have easier labors with fewer C-sections and deliver healthier, more alert babies. About a decade ago, the American College of Obstetrics and Gynecology lifted its cautions on exercising during pregnancy. Always inform your doctor of your exercise program, but most likely you can basically keep doing what you've been doing as long as you haven't been overexercising (no more than five times a week for 60 minutes!), don't experience any abdominal cramping or pain, check your diastasis before doing any crunches (after the first trimester, most women find that their gap is too wide for crunches), and you're careful about dehydration and heat exhaustion.

7. **Drink plenty of water.** At least eight glasses a day will help prevent dehydration and heat exhaustion, especially if you live in a hotter climate. But even if you reside in Alaska, you still need six to eight glasses of water to increase your blood volume and deliver nutrients to your baby.

8. **Eat small, frequent meals.** At the beginning of your pregnancy, it will help with morning sickness, and at the end of your preg-

nancy it will help with fatigue and heartburn. With your uterus pushing your stomach up and squishing it against your diaphragm and lungs, you won't be able to fit much more than a small meal in there anyway.

9. **Eat a well-balanced diet.** The University of Maine at Orono recently found that the majority of pregnant women are falling short on important nutrients such as folic acid, iron, calcium, and some B vitamins. To get all the nutrients you need, make sure you take your prenatal vitamins and eat a variety of foods from all the food groups. You need at least two to three servings of protein, three to four servings of dairy products, five to nine servings of fruits and vegetables, and six to nine servings of grains. If you're a vegetarian, you need to pay extra attention to the foods you're eating to make sure you're meeting your protein and vitamin B12 requirements (FYI—if you're hoping for a girl, vegetarians are 20 percent more likely to deliver a female). And if you have any confusion or concerns with this pregnancy, go to the expert, a registered dietitian, who can help you design a healthy pregnancy diet to suit your needs.

10. **Don't worry about postpartum weight loss.** It will be much easier to outsmart your postpartum fat cells this time around because you already have the knowledge and tools from reading this book. Just open it again after you've delivered, to put on the finishing touches.

There is one exception to number ten—forty-plus-year-old pregnancies. If you're forty or over, I'm not telling you to start worrying about postpartum weight loss—just to be aware of the fact that there's a good chance you'll go straight from the maternity ward into perimenopause. And perimenopausal fat cells are even stronger and more stubborn than postpartum ones. I apologize for being the bearer of bad fat-cell news, but here's some research that might help make you feel better: Women who have babies in their forties are more likely to be alive for their one-hundredth birthday. So, in the long run, you get a longer life. In the short run, you get more stubborn fat cells.

FROM POSTPARTUM TO PERIMENOPAUSE: PREPARING FOR YOUR NEXT STAGE OF PASSAGE

An expanding waistline, stubborn fat cells, weight gain, night sweats, hot flashes, memory loss, mood swings, depression, confusion, fatigue—it sounds so similar to the postpartum period because it is. Dropping estrogen levels are behind all the changes we experience during both the postpartum months and the perimenopausal years. The difference with perimenopause is that it will last for the next ten years instead of a few months. And the difference with perimenopausal fat cells is that they will take longer to outsmart.

Whether you go directly from postpartum into perimenopause, or you're still in your twenties and have another decade or so to go before it blindsides you, I want to help you to gain a full understanding and appreciation of the body changes that occur: why all of a sudden, you can't zip up your jeans (but you swear you could yesterday); why your stomach is starting to look like it's three months pregnant again (but your husband had a vasectomy); why your bra is so tight that it leaves indents in your skin (but you just bought it last week); and why you can't seem to lose the weight no matter how hard you try (but you're exercising and eating right). As with everything that happens in a woman's body, there is a biological explanation.

When your fat cells detect a slightly lower estrogen reading that signals the beginning of your ten-plus-year perimenopausal transition, they come to your aid to start to produce estrogen for you. It's one of their highly evolved functions to ease your transition and help you live a long and healthy life. They know that eventually your ovaries will stop producing estrogen, so they start preparing to take over the ovaries' job by increasing their size, number, and fat-storing ability. Interestingly enough, the fat cells in your waist, abdomen, breasts, and back grow the largest because they are better equipped to produce estrogen than the fat cells in your buttocks, hips, and thighs. The larger and more active your upper-body fat cells become, the more estrogen will be produced, and the more benefits you will receive: fewer hot flashes, milder mood swings, improved sleep, a reduced risk of osteoporosis, a healthier heart, and an overall easier transition. This is why larger women have always reported less menopausal stress, while leaner women have the most difficulty with the transition. This is why your body is programmed to gain about ten pounds of fat and expand your waist by two inches. This is why fifty million women are crying out for help this very minute.

As with the postpartum period, dieting is *not* the answer to that cry for help. When we wage war against our fat cells during midlife, they fight back with a vengeance and grow even larger. But there is an effective solution: *Your Postpartum Peace Plan is also your Perimenopausal Peace Plan.* The same strategies you've been following to outsmart postbaby fat will also shrink your perimenopausal fat cells without compromising their ability to produce estrogen and enhance your well-being. Smaller portions, smaller meals, more frequent meals, staying away from dieting, and exercising sixty minutes four to five days a week (the upper end of the exercise recommendation) will keep your menopausal fat cells in check. As long as you continue with basically the same eating and exercising strategies you're doing right now, you'll successfully manage your midlife weight gain. A recent study published in the journal *Menopause* found that lifestyle can override biology; and exercise (or lack of it), in particular, was the biggest determining factor in how much weight women gained during the menopausal transition. There's that e-word again. If you haven't already, it's time to wake up and smell the sweaty socks. *Exercise is your solution to everything—a vital pregnancy, a svelte postpartum body, and a fit menopause.*

As you reach this important stage in your female lifecycle, my best advice is to arm yourself with knowledge. Ask questions, talk about it, and read about it. There are hundreds of books available to help you through the perimenopausal transition, and I wrote one of them, *Outsmarting the Midlife Fat Cell,* to help you manage your midlife weight crisis with understanding and action. The more knowledge, understanding, and skills you acquire, the more likely you'll journey through the rest of your life trimmer, healthier, happier, and calmer.

LIFE AFTER BIRTH: KIDS, CHAOS, AND THE TRICKLE-DOWN EFFECT

"Is there life after birth?" asked Kim as she rushed into my office twenty minutes late with a diaper bag over her arm, spit up in her hair, and oatmeal on her shirt. "My babysitter was late, my husband's on a business trip, my baby discovered that oatmeal sticks to the wall if it's thrown hard enough, and my son forgot his homework so I had to drop it off to him at school. I didn't have time to shower or change, and I grabbed the diaper bag instead of my purse so I couldn't even brush my hair or put lipstick on in the car. I'm a mess! I don't have the time to take care of my body, and I feel like I'm losing my mind. If I were to have an IQ test right now, I'm convinced the results would come back negative. Forget life after death; I'm wondering if there is such a thing as *life after birth.*"

Kim and I concluded that there is indeed life after birth—a life full of diaper rashes, temper tantrums, terrible twos, T-ball, soccer games, swim lessons, science projects, piano recitals, homework, birthday parties, sibling rivalry, bed-wetting, food fights, dirty cars, messy houses, and unwashed hair. And in a few years, a life full of ornery adolescents, not-so-sweet sixteens, sex education, dances, dating, driver's licenses, drug and alcohol worries, college applications, and marriage licenses. I think you'll agree, *motherhood isn't just a full-time job; it's a lifetime adventure.*

During these next six years and beyond, your life will be filled with unavoidable changes, unending challenges, and unrelenting chaos that may throw you off-kilter and make you question your ability to stay healthy, fit, and sane. For some of you, the day-to-day whirlwind of being a mother already greets you every morning with multiple lunches to pack, mouths to feed, bodies to dress, homework to organize, and car pools to coordinate. If you haven't already found yourself stressed to the max with motherhood, one or all of the following scenarios is bound to come between you and the Postpartum Peace Plan:

- You'll be feeling confident about your body one day, and the next day you're dropping off your "baby" for his first day of kindergarten with tears in your eyes . . . when all of a sudden, you spot her—that twenty-five-year-old "skinny mini" with a to-die-for body, puffed hair, and perfectly applied makeup who makes you look like you could be *her* mother. With your tearful thoughts now turned away from "your baby growing up" to "you're growing old," you rush home, stand in front of the mirror obsessing about your matronly looking body, and start calling the diet programs and plastic surgeons in the yellow pages.

- You'll be feeling consistent with your eating one day, and the next day the Girl Scout cookies show up, followed by the Valentine's candy, Easter eggs, jelly beans, Halloween candy, Christmas cookies, cotton candy, and gummy bears. As your kids grow up, foods you never thought you'd keep in the house suddenly appear—and since "stressed" spelled backward is "desserts," you devour their treats in reckless abandon.

- You'll be feeling fit one day, and the next day all three kids come home from school sick, then you get the flu, then your husband comes down with it (who is a worse patient than all three kids combined), and before you know it, a month has gone down the tube with no exercise, and you feel like you've blown it.

You haven't blown it. There is no blowing the Postpartum Peace Plan. In the scope of your lifetime commitment to outsmarting your postbaby fat cells, it doesn't matter if you can't exercise for a few weeks, if you binge on your kid's jelly beans during a stress breakdown, or if you go through a bout of body dissatisfaction. These temporary glitches are a part of life, and particularly a part of a mother's life. Anticipate them, prepare yourself for them, and don't wait until "things calm down" to renew your commitment to exercising and eating moderately—you'll be waiting eighteen years. Instead, acknowledge your hectic schedule, time restraints, and stressful life—and do whatever you can to keep your body healthy and your fat cells outsmarted.

As time goes on and you continue with the Postpartum Peace Plan, you won't have to consciously do anything to keep your body healthy because it stops being a plan and becomes the way you live. You'll automatically want to find a way to fit exercise into your "week from hell" because you know you need it more than ever to keep your sanity. You'll strive to fuel your body with small meals because you know you need the energy to get the fifty items on your to-do list done. And you'll make a point of doing something every day to take care of your body because you respect and cherish it—and want to teach your children to do the same.

By living the Postpartum Peace Plan, the added bonus is that you'll automatically be passing down healthy behaviors to your children, and encouraging them by your example to move, feed, and respect their bodies. It's what I call the Trickle-Down Effect, and recent research has shown just how important this legacy is:

- If you exercise, your children will be more likely to value fitness.
- If you eat fruits and vegetables, they will be more likely to follow in your produce-loving footsteps.
- If you drink milk, they will be more likely to opt for dairy over diet soft drinks.

- If you eat a wide variety of foods in moderation, they will be more likely to fuel their bodies with moderate portions.
- If you maintain a healthy weight, they will be more likely to keep their bodies fit and healthy.
- If you give up dieting, they will be more likely to never start.
- If you have a positive body image, they will be more likely to look in the mirror with a smile.

Your children need you to be healthy and trickle down your healthy behaviors to them. Over the past forty years, the incidence of childhood obesity has increased by 50 percent, the number of dieting girls has risen by a staggering 1300 percent, and the incidence of adolescent eating disorders has tripled. Every mother I know is terrified by these statistics and wants to do everything she can to save her children from the dangers of dieting, eating disorders, and obesity. Are you? By living the Postpartum Peace Plan, you already are protecting your children. *You're modeling a healthy relationship with food and your body, and thereby creating a safe haven in your home to help balance the persuasive media messages and peer pressure to diet and pursue thinness.*

Before reading this book, you may have been weight-preoccupied, obsessed with dieting, and caught in a downward spiral of body dissatisfaction. What would you have taught your children if you didn't become a nondieting, body-accepting mother? That women are supposed to diet and be at war with their bodies? That it's normal to deprive your body of nourishment? That it's acceptable female behavior to wake up every morning hating your body? Research has found that daughters, in particular, pay very close attention to the spoken and unspoken messages mothers give about food, fat, weight, and the female body.

- Researchers at Stanford University School of Medicine found that over half of sixth grade girls learned about dieting from their mothers.

- According to the results of a study at Wesleyan University, mothers who diet are two-and-one-half times more likely to encourage their daughters to restrict their eating.
- A Pennsylvania State University study found that the mother–daughter diet connection can begin as early as age five. If the mothers dieted, their five-year-old daughters were twice as likely to have thoughts about dieting.
- Yale University researchers found that eating disorders are strongly passed from mother to daughter and from generation to generation.

If you have a daughter at home and want more guidance to help her (and you) break free from the dieting industry, society's thin ideal, body dissatisfaction, and eating disorders, I highly suggest that you read another of my books, *Outsmarting the Mother–Daughter Food Trap*. It is a potentially lifesaving manual that encourages mothers and daughters of all ages to turn their backs on dieting and work together to feed and respect the bodies they were born with.

Life after birth may be chaotic and difficult to manage at times, but your life is more important now than it's ever been. You are a mother, and that makes you a life skills teacher, mentor, and role model. Think of the saying, "The apple doesn't fall far from the tree." If the tree is healthy, vibrant, well nourished, and strong rooted—its fruit will be, too. If you want your children to be healthy, fit, and self-assured, you have to be healthy, fit, and self-assured first. In essence, *we need to become the children we want to raise*. And from the thousands of mothers that I've counseled and interviewed, this trickle-down effect has been one of the most powerful motivators to keeping the Postpartum Peace Plan a part of their lives forever.

Growing, Growing, Gone: Outsmarting Your Fat Cells Forever

My goal in writing this book was to help you outsmart your fat cells in the postpartum months, but as you now know, it's also your manual for outsmarting your fat cells throughout your life and helping your children to outsmart theirs in a positive, nondieting, body-accepting way. Therefore, the Postpartum Peace Plan doesn't stop when you lose your pregnancy weight, it continues for the rest of your life—and works for the rest of your life. A number of studies from the United States, Sweden, and elsewhere have followed postpartum women over time to discover what separated the weight loss maintainers from the regainers. Those women who successfully maintained their weight loss:

- didn't diet (of course);
- exercised regularly (of course again), with walking as their most common activity;
- ate three small meals and two snacks a day;
- ate their favorite foods;
- didn't cut the fat out of their diets; and
- ate more fruits and vegetables.

So, there you have it from women around the world—the secrets to losing postbaby pounds and the scientific proof for the Postpartum Peace Plan. It's not rocket science, and it's not sensational enough to make the ten o'clock evening news, *but this is what it takes to successfully and permanently outsmart your postpartum fat cells.*

How do you know when you've successfully outsmarted your postpartum fat cells? You'll know, but it won't be the scale that informs you. Reaching your exact prepregnancy weight doesn't define success. Some of you will weigh a few pounds more, and others will weigh forty pounds less (if you were overweight and out of shape before you got pregnant). Fitting into a weight chart or wearing a size six doesn't define success either, neither does losing more weight than your friend, or weighing less than your mother did after she had you.

So, what does define success? Reaching a comfortable, fit, healthy weight that's right for you. A weight that moves around freely, runs up three flights of stairs without getting out of breath, feels confident wearing a bathing suit in public, cuddles your baby and caresses your partner, doesn't have to live on lettuce leaves to sustain itself, and is free of weight-related medical problems such as high blood pressure, high blood cholesterol, and high blood sugar. *That's the definition of a healthy, successful weight—even if it falls above your recommended weight for height or it's a few pounds above where you want to be.*

With this new definition, do you feel like you've successfully outsmarted your postpartum fat cells? Or perhaps you are dying to turn the table and pose that same question to me. Have I been successful? Has the Postpartum Peace Plan worked for its originator? Has the Fat Cell Lady outsmarted her own? By my definition of success, I respond with a resounding YES! I am at a comfortable, confident, fit, healthy weight. I have personally followed everything that I've recommended to you. I've been consistent with exercise three times a week and moderate in my eating every day of the week. I've pampered myself, gotten the support I need, calmed myself down about hair loss, and embraced my body every step of the way. Where has it gotten me? To exactly where I want to be—fit, healthy, energetic, confident, and happy. Not to the exact weight I was before I got pregnant, but to the exact level of fitness and body appreciation that I aspired to.

As you know, I don't weigh myself, but for you Doubting Theresas out there, I got on the scale this morning at my doctor's office, and the number 128 stared back at me. It didn't affect me one way or the other. I was neither tickled pink nor turning blue; I just took it at face value and said, "Oh, that means I must have lost about 35 pounds since I've had Tyler. And since I don't know what my exact weight was before I got pregnant, my guess is that I'm about three or four pounds higher." The average weight retained for those women who exercise is about three pounds, so it made sense that, as an exercising woman, I was about average.

But it took me over a year to get to that "average," and I've written this book as I have personally gone through the postpartum time line outlined for you. I began writing leisurely at six weeks postpartum, and scribbled frantically trying to meet my deadline at sixteen months. I've had the same ups and downs, wonders and worries, adjustments and frustrations as you've had. But I never lost faith in my body or doubted my knowledge and ability to lose weight in a healthy way. And it paid off, because I've made peace with my postpartum body and have successfully outsmarted my postpartum fat cells. It is my sincere hope that you have (or will soon) too—and will keep them outsmarted forever.

What's Your Postpartum Peace Plan for the Next Six Years?

At this point you know what to do: Check all the strategies that you'll use to continue outsmarting your postpartum fat cells—and keep them outsmarted forever.

What Will You Do to Pamper Yourself?

___ I will continue to think positively about my body and its ability to lose weight.

___ I will continue to pamper my body with baths, massages, facials, manicures, and anything else that makes me feel good.

___ I will realize that my body needs to be taken care of throughout my life.

What Will You Do to Eat Moderately With a Regular Meal Schedule?

___ I will be consistent with my eating-habit changes, focusing on eating moderate portions and small, frequent meals.

___ If I decide to have another child, I will make sure that I take my prenatal vitamins, trust my food cravings, and eat a well-balanced diet.

___ I will pass on healthy, moderate, nondieting eating behaviors to my children.

What Will You Do to Actively Move Your Body?

___ I will be consistent with my aerobic-exercise program, weight lifting, and crunches.

___ For a fat-burning boost, I will add another day of exercise, a new activity, and/or five, ten, or fifteen minutes to my aerobic exercise sessions.

___ I will not overexercise—sixty minutes, five times a week is the most I'll do.

___ I will get right back into my exercise program if uncontrollable circumstances of my hectic life as a mother get in the way.

___ I will model an active lifestyle for my children.

What Will You Do to Calm Your Stress?

___ I will realize that the last few pounds are the most difficult to lose, and will give myself another three to six months to lose them.

___ When I enter perimenopause, I will arm myself with knowledge and gain an understanding of the many changes that go along with "the change."

____ I will prepare myself for the chaos of motherhood, realizing that the Postpartum Peace Plan can withstand the stress and help to minimize it.

What Will You Do to Embrace Your New Body?

____ I will acknowledge that pregnancy changed my body for the better, making it healthier by reducing my risk of breast and ovarian cancers, increasing my bone density, and enhancing my longevity and happiness.

____ I will define success by reaching a comfortable, healthy weight that's right for me.

____ I will accept and respect my body, and by example, teach my children to accept and respect theirs.

____ I will acknowledge the positive changes in my body, and keep the Postpartum Peace Plan a part of my life forever.

You're at the end of this book, and although I'd love to continue giving you support by taking you through the next six decades, you won't need it. The knowledge and skills you've learned and the lifestyle changes you've made will benefit you for the rest of your life. Your exercise program will keep you mobile, strong, and fit; your moderate eating habits will keep you vital, healthy, and trim; and your commitment to taking care of yourself will keep you balanced, relaxed, and self-assured for decades to come. The Postpartum Peace Plan may have been designed for the months and years following birth, but it is destined to become your life-enhancing, fat-burning, muscle-building, body image–boosting, stress-reducing, mood-balancing, sanity-saving program forever.

If you read through this entire book in a night, a week, or a month, go back to chapter 4 and start at the beginning of the Postpartum Peace Plan. You may have all the knowledge about your stubborn postpartum fat cells, but following the specific steps of the PEACE Plan is what it takes to outsmart them. If you've been committed to the program as outlined and have given your body permission to lose weight on its own schedule, I sincerely hope that you have made peace with your fat cells, food intake, fitness level, and female body—and have found unprecedented success by reading this book, because it was written for you. Congratulations on your baby, and congratulations on outsmarting your female fat cells after having your baby! I wish you continued happiness and success, and all the best that life has to offer.

Additional Resources

THE POSTPARTUM PEACE PLAN PERSONAL EATING JOURNAL

Food records have been strongly suggested as an effective and necessary tool for changing eating behaviors, and the *Postpartum Peace Plan Personal Eating Journal* makes this important tool simple, easy, and convenient. Small enough to fit into your purse or briefcase, it contains 180 days of food records, plus additional exercise records and tip sheets to successfully outsmart your postbaby fat cells. To order this companion to success please visit the www.waterhousepublications.com website or send $8 plus $2 shipping and handling to:

Waterhouse Publications
P.O. Box 4735
Portland, ME 04112

WORKBOOKS AND OTHER PUBLICATIONS

For a complete listing of other books, journals, and workbooks by Debra Waterhouse, as well as other materials helpful in changing eating and exercise habits, again please visit the www.waterhousepublications.com website or write to the above address for a brochure.

Seminars & Workshops

If your organization is interested in a presentation on *Outsmarting the Female Fat Cell—After Pregnancy* or other women's health topic, please contact:

Debra Waterhouse
PMB 342
6114 LaSalle Avenue
Oakland, CA 94611

Suggested Reading

Because new mothers are often eager for information, I have attempted to provide a comprehensive reading list on postpartum care, including pregnancy books with a significant "after-the-baby" section as well as general weight-loss and child-feeding books with a nonrestrictive approach. Although I may not agree with everything the authors recommend, each of the following books has some valuable information to offer.

Barrett, N. *I Wish Someone Had Told Me: The Realistic Guide to Early Motherhood.* New York: Fireside, 1997.

Behan, E. *Eat Well, Lose Weight While Breastfeeding.* New York: Villard, 1992.

———. *The Pregnancy Diet.* New York: Pocket, 1999.

Berman, C., and Jacki Fromer. *Meals Without Squeals, Teaching Children About Food.* Palo Alto: Bull Publishing, 1997.

Boltow, M. K. *The Third Shift: Managing Hard Choices in Our Careers, Houses and Lives as Women.* San Francisco: Jossey-Bass, 2000.

Borysenko, J. *A Woman's Book of Life.* New York: Riverhead, 1996.

Carter, L., with L. S. Ostrow. *The Miracle Year: An Expectant Parent's Guide to the Miraculous Six Months Before—and After—the Birth of Their First Baby.* New York: Pocket, 1991.

Clapp, J. F. *Exercising Through Your Pregnancy.* Champaign, Ill.: Human Kinetics, 1998.

Dougherty, K., and G. Gaesser. *The Spark.* New York: Fawcett Columbine, 1996.

Duff, S. *The Post-Pregnancy Diet.* New York: Signet, 1989.

Dunnewold, A., and D. Sanford. *Postpartum Survival Guide.* Oakland, Calif.: New Harbinger, 1994.

Eastman, M. *Taming the Dragon in Your Child.* New York: Wiley, 1994.

Editors of *Fitness* magazine with Ginny Graves. *Pregnancy Fitness.* New York: Three Rivers Press, 1999.

Editors of *Working Mother* magazine. *The Working Mother Book of Time.* New York: St. Martin's, 2000.

Eisenberg, A., H. Murkoff, and S. Hathaway. *What to Expect When You're Expecting.* New York: Workman, 1984.

———. *What to Expect the First Year.* New York: Workman, 1989.

Fisher, H. *The First Sex.* New York: Random House, 1999.

Gore, A. *The Hip Mama Survival Guide.* New York: Hyperion, 1998.

———. *The Mother Trip.* Seattle: Seal Press, 2000.

Haffner, D. W. *From Diapers to Dating.* New York: Newmarket Press, 1999.

Hall, L. *Full Lives: Women Who Have Freed Themselves from Weight Obsessions.* Carlsbad, Calif.: Gurze Books, 1993.

Hirschmann, J. R., and C. H. Munter. *Overcoming Overeating.* New York: Fawcett Columbine, 1988.

———. *When Women Stop Hating Their Bodies.* New York: Fawcett Columbine, 1995.

Hochschild, A. R. *The Time Bind.* New York: Henry Holt, 1997.

Huysman, A. *A Mother's Tears.* New York: Seven Stories Press, 1998.

Iovine, V. *The Girlfriend's Guide to Pregnancy.* New York: Pocket, 1995.

———. *The Girlfriend's Guide to Surviving the First Year of Motherhood.* New York: Berkley, 1997.

———. *The Girlfriend's Guide to Toddlers.* New York: Berkley, 1999.

Kano, S. *Making Peace with Food.* New York: Perennial Library, 1989.

Kitzinger, S. *The Year After Childbirth.* New York: Fireside, 1996.

Kleiman, K., and V. Raskin. *This Isn't What I Expected.* New York: Bantam, 1994.

Levine, M. J. *I Wish I Were Thin, I Wish I Were Fat.* New York: Vanderbilt Press, 1997.

Maas, J. B. *Power Sleep.* New York: Villard, 1998.

Maushart, S. *The Mask of Motherhood.* New York: Penguin, 1999.

Mellin, L. *The Solution: Winning Ways to Permanent Weight Loss.* New York: Regan Books, 1997.

Mitchell, S., and C. Christie. *I'd Kill for a Cookie: A Simple Six-Week Plan to Conquer Stress Eating.* New York: Dutton, 1997.

Murphy, J. *Baby Tips for New Moms: First 4 Months.* Tucson: Fisher Books, 1998.

Nelson, M. *Strong Women Stay Young.* New York: Bantam, 1997.

Newmark, G. *How to Raise Emotionally Healthy Children.* Tarzana, Calif.: NMI Publishers, 1999.

Northrup, C. *Women's Bodies, Women's Wisdom.* New York: Bantam, 1998.

Orenstein, P. *Flux.* New York: Doubleday, 2000.

Peeke, P. *Fight Fat After Forty.* New York: Viking, 2000.

Placksin, S. *Mothering the New Mother.* New York: Newmarket Press, 2000.

Pryor, G. *Nursing Mother, Working Mother.* Boston: Harvard Common Press, 1997.

Reichman, J. *I'm Not in the Mood.* New York: Morrow, 1998.

Roan, S. *Our Daughters' Health.* New York: Hyperion, 2001.

Roche, L. *Meditation Made Easy.* San Francisco: Harper, 1998.

Roth, G. *Feeding the Hungry Heart.* Indianapolis: Bobbs-Merrill, 1982.

———. *Breaking Free from Compulsive Overeating.* Indianapolis: Bobbs-Merrill, 1984.

———. *When Food Is Love.* New York: Dutton, 1991.

———. *Appetites.* New York: Dutton, 1996.

———. *When You Eat at the Refrigerator, Pull Up a Chair.* New York: Hyperion, 1998.

Satter, E. *Child of Mine.* Palo Alto: Bull Publishing, 1986.

———. *How to Get Your Kid to Eat . . . But Not Too Much.* Palo Alto: Bull Publishing, 1987.

———. *Secrets of Feeding a Healthy Family.* Madison, Wis.: Kelcy Press, 1999.

Sears, W., and M. Sears. *300 Questions New Parents Ask: About Pregnancy, Childbirth, and Infant and Child Care.* New York: Plume, 1991.

Small, M. *Our Babies, Ourselves: How Biology and Culture Shape the Way We Parent.* New York: Anchor, 1998.

Somer, E. *Nutrition for Women.* New York: Henry Holt, 1993.

———. *The Origin Diet.* New York: Henry Holt, 2001.

Sweeney, J. *I Know I Should Exercise, But . . .* San Diego: Pacific Valley Press, 1998.

Tamopolsky, M. *Gender Differences in Metabolism: Practical and Nutritional Implications.* New York: CRC Press, 1998.

Tribole, E. *Stealth Health.* New York: Viking, 1998.

Tribole, E., and E. Resch. *Intuitive Eating.* New York: St. Martin's, 1995.

Trindade, E., and V. Shaw, PhD. *Strollercize: The Workout for New Mothers.* New York: Three Rivers Press, 2001.

Tuper, J. *Maternal Fitness.* New York: Simon and Schuster, 1999.

Waggoner, G., and D. Stumpf. *From Baby to Bikini.* New York: Warner, 1999.

Ward, E. *Pregnancy Nutrition: Good Health for You and Your Baby.* New York: Wiley, 1998.

Waterhouse, D. *Outsmarting the Midlife Fat Cell.* New York: Hyperion, 1998.

———. *Outsmarting the Female Fat Cell.* New York: Hyperion, 1999.

———. *Outsmarting Female Fatigue.* New York: Hyperion, 2001.

———. *Outsmarting the Mother–Daughter Food Trap.* New York: Hyperion, 2001.

———. *Outsmarting Female Food Cravings.* New York: Hyperion, 2002.

Bibliography

"A. M. Good News." *Environmental Nutrition* 20(1997): 3.

Abramovitz, B. A., et al. "Five-Year-Old Girls' Ideas About Dieting Are Predicted by Their Mothers' Dieting." *Journal of the American Dietetic Association* 100 (2000): 1157.

Adair, L. S., et al. "Feeding Babies: Mothers' Decisions in an Urban U.S. Setting." *Medical Anthropology* 17 (1983): 1.

Affonso, D. "Postpartum Depression: A Nursing Perspective on Women's Health and Behaviors." *Images Journal of Nursing Scholarship* 24 (1992): 215.

Alder, E., et al. "The Relationship Between Breast-Feeding Persistence, Sexuality and Mood in Postpartum Women." *Psychological Medicine* 18 (1988): 389.

Allen, R. E., et al. "Pelvic Floor Damage and Childbirth: A Neuropsychological Study." *British Journal of Obstetrics and Gynecology* 99 (1992): 724.

Andersen, R. E., et al. "Changes in Bone Mineral Content in Obese Dieting Women." *Metabolism: Clinical and Experimental* 46 (1997): 857.

Appleby, P. N., et al. "Low Body Mass Index in Non-Meat Eaters: The Possible Roles of Animal Fat, Dietary Fibre and Alcohol." *International Journal of Obesity and Related Metabolic Disorders* 22 (1998): 454.

Areias, M., et al. "Comparative Incidence of Depression in Women and Men, During Pregnancy and After Childbirth." *British Journal of Psychiatry* 169 (1996): 30.

Aronoff, N. J., et al. "Gender and Body Mass Index as Related to the Night-Eating Syndrome in Obese Outpatients." *Journal of the American Dietetic Association* 101 (2001): 102.

Asp, K. "Run, Mama, Run." *Shape Presents Fit Pregnancy,* Winter 1999, p. 26.

Astrup, A., et al. "Meta-Analysis of Resting Metabolic Rate in Formerly Obese Subjects." *American Journal of Clinical Nutrition* 69 (1999): 1117.

Ballew, C., et al. "Nutrient Intakes and Dietary Patterns of Young Children by Dietary Fat Intakes." *Journal of Pediatrics* 136 (2000): 181.

Barash, I., et al. "Leptin Is a Metabolic Signal to the Reproductive System." *Endocrinology* 137 (1996): 3144.

Barr, S. I., et al. "Energy Intakes Are Higher During the Luteal Phase of Ovulatory Menstrual Cycles." *American Journal of Clinical Nutrition* 61 (1995): 39.

Bates, C. D. "Why You Should Be an Optimist." *Shape,* October 2000, p. 144.

"Battling the Blues." *American Health,* September 1999, p. 14.

Beck, C. T. "Screening Methods for Postpartum Depression." *Journal of Obstetrics, Gynecological, and Neonatal Nursing* 24 (1995): 308.

Behan, E. 1999. *The Pregnancy Diet.* New York: Pocket.

Bek, K. M., et al. "Risk of Anal Incontinence from Subsequent Vaginal Delivery After a Complete Anal Sphincter Tear." *British Journal of Obstetrics and Gynecology* 99 (1992): 724.

Blais, M. A., et al. "Pregnancy: Outcome and Impact on Symptomatology in a Cohort of Eating-Disordered Women." *International Journal of Eating Disorders* 27 (2000): 140.

Blumenthal, J. A., et al. "Exercise and Weight Loss Reduce Blood Pressure in Men and Women with Mild Hypertension." *Archives of Internal Medicine* 160 (2000): 1947.

Boardley, D. J., et al. "The Relationship Between Diet, Activity, and Other Factors, and Postpartum Weight Change by Race." *Obstetrics and Gynecology* 86 (1995): 834.

Borysenko, J. 1996. *A Woman's Book of Life.* New York: Riverhead.

"Breast-Feeding as an Antidote to Stress." *Self,* August 1999, p. 110.

Brewer, M. M., et al. "Postpartum Changes in Maternal Weight and Body Fat Depots in Lactating vs. Nonlactating Women." *American Journal of Clinical Nutrition* 49 (1989): 259.

Bro, R., et al. "Effects of a Breakfast Program on On-Task Behaviors of Vocational High School Students." *Journal of Educational Research* 90 (1996): 111.

Brody, L. "1999 Body Image Survey Results." *Shape,* June 1999, p. 150.

Bronstein, M. N., et al. "Unexpected Relationship Between Fat Mass and Basal Metabolic Rate in Pregnant Women." *British Journal of Nutrition* 75 (1996): 659.

Brown, J. E., et al. "Nutrition and Multifetal Pregnancy." *Journal of the American Dietetic Association* 100 (2000): 3.

Butte, N. F., et al. "Body Composition Changes During Lactation Are Highly Variable Among Women." *Journal of Nutrition* 128 (1998): 381S.

———. "Adjustments in Energy Expenditure and Substrate Utilization During Late Pregnancy and Lactation." *American Journal of Clinical Nutrition* 69 (1999): 299.

Campbell, S. B., et al. "Prevalence and Correlates of Postpartum Depression in First-Time Mothers." *Journal of Abnormal Psychology* 100 (1991): 594.

Campbell, W. W., et al. "Energy Requirement for Long-Term Body Weight Maintenance in Older Women." *Metabolism: Clinical and Experimental* 46 (1997): 884.

Carper, J. L., et al. "Young Girls' Emerging Dietary Restraint and Disinhibition Are Related to Parental Control in Child Feeding." *Appetite* 35 (2000): 121.

Cash, T. F., et al. "The Great American Shape Up." *Psychology Today,* April 11, 1986, p. 30.

Chaliha, C., et al. "Antenatal Prediction of Postpartum Urinary and Fecal Incontinence." *Obstetrics and Gynecology* 94(1999): 689.

Chambers, E. "Cognitive Strategies for Reporting Portion Sizes Using Dietary Recall Procedures." *Journal of the American Dietetic Association* 100 (2000): 891.

Chapman, D. J., et al. "Identification of Risk Factors for Delayed Onset of Lactation." *Journal of the American Dietetic Association* 99 (1999): 450.

"Chew on This." *UC Berkeley Wellness Letter,* April 2000, p. 8.

Clark, M., et al. "The Impact of Pregnancy on Eating Behaviour and Aspects of Weight Concern." *International Journal of Obesity* 23 (1999): 18.

Colino, S., et al. "Sounding Off About Noise." *American Health for Women,* October 1998, p. 64.

Conway, D. L., et al. "Effects of New Criteria for Type 2 Diabetes on the Rate of Postpartum Glucose Intolerance in Women with Gestational Diabetes." *American Journal of Obstetrics and Gynecology* 181 (1999): 610.

Cooper, K. N. "Upon Arrival, What Happens in the Hospital They Whisk Your Baby Away." *Shape Presents Fit Pregnancy,* August/September 2000, p. 64.

Copper, T. L., et al. "The Relationship of Maternal Attitude Toward Weight Gain to Weight Gain During Pregnancy and Low Birth Weight." *Obstetrics and Gynecology* 85 (1995): 590.

Corral, M., et al. "Bright Light Therapy's Effect on Postpartum Depression." *American Journal of Psychiatry* 157 (2000): 303.

Cox, J., et al. "Detection of Postnatal Depression: Development of the 10-Item Edinburgh Post-Natal Depression Scale." *British Journal of Psychiatry* 150 (1987): 782.

Crowell, D. T. "Weight Change in the Postpartum Period." *Journal of Nurse-Midwifery* 40 (1995): 418.

Dam, J. K. L., et al. "Searching for the Perfect Body." *People,* September 4, 2000, pp. 114–122.

Davies, K., et al. "Body Image and Dieting in Pregnancy." *Journal of Psychosomatic Research* 38 (1994): 787.

de Bruin, N. C., et al. "Energy Utilization and Growth in Breast-Fed and Formula-Fed Infants Measured Prospectively During the First Year of Life." *American Journal of Clinical Nutrition* 67 (1998): 885.

Devine, C. M., et al. "Women's Perceptions About the Way Social Roles Promote or Constrain Personal Nutrition Care." *Women and Health* 19 (1992): 79.

———. "Maternal Weight-Loss Patterns During Prolonged Lactation." *American Journal of Clinical Nutrition* 58 (1993): 162.

———. "A Randomized Study of the Effects of Aerobic Exercise by Lactating Women on Breast-Milk Volume and Composition." *The New England Journal of Medicine* 330 (1994): 449.

———. "Continuity and Change in Women's Weight Orientations and Lifestyle Practices Through Pregnancy and the Postpartum Period: The Influence of Life Course Trajectories and Transitional Events." *Social Science and Medicine* 50 (2000): 567.

"Dietary Variety Loses Favor as Nutritionists Find It Causes Weight Gain." *Tufts University Health and Nutrition Letter,* July 1999, p. 4.

"Do Any Weight-Loss Supplements Work, Ever?" *Women's Health Advisor,* May 2000, p. 6.

Dohney, K. "Feeding Facts, the Latest News and Views on the Best Formula for Your Baby." *Shape Presents Fit Pregnancy,* February/March 2000, p. 60.

Donnelly, V. S., et al. "Obstetric Events Leading to Anal Sphincter Damage." *Obstetrics and Gynecology* 92 (1998): 955.

Doran, L., et al. "Energy and Nutrient Inadequacies in the Diets of Low-Income Women Who Breast-Feed." *Journal of the American Dietetic Association* 97 (1997): 1283.

Duff, S. 1989. *The Post-Pregnancy Diet.* New York: Signet.

Dugdale, A. E., et al. "The Effect of Lactation and Other Factors on Post-Partum Changes in Body-Weight and Triceps Skinfold Thickness." *British Journal of Nutrition* 61 (1989): 149.

Dunn Bates, C., et al. "Why We're So Dissatisfied with Sex." *Shape,* December 1999, p. 30.

Dusdieker, L. B., et al. "Is Milk Production Impaired by Dieting During Lactation?" *American Journal of Clinical Nutrition* 59 (1994): 833.

Dwyer, J. T., et al. "Prevalence of Marked Overweight and Obesity in a Multiethnic Pediatric Population: Findings from the Child and Adolescent Trial for Cardiovascular Health (CATCH) Study." *Journal of the American Dietetic Association* 100 (2000): 1149.

Eastman, M. 1994. *Taming the Dragon in Your Child.* New York:Wiley.

"Easy Way to Ease Anxiety." *Shape,* June 1999, p. 28.

"Eat Fat, Get Thin?" *UC Berkeley Wellness Letter,* April 2000, p. 1.

"Eat More Often to Combat Overeating." *Environmental Nutrition,* April 2000, p. 8.

Eck Clemens, L. H., et al. "The Effect of Eating Out on Quality of Diet in Premenopausal Women." *Journal of the American Dietetic Association* 99 (1999): 442.

Eidelman, A., et al. "Postpartum Cognitive Deficits: Cognitive Deficits in Women After Childbirth." *Obstetrics and Gynecology* 81 (1993): 764.

Eisenberg, A., et al. 1984. *What to Expect When You're Expecting.* New York: Workman.

———. 1989. *What to Expect the First Year.* New York: Workman.

Fairburn, C. G., et al. "The Impact of Pregnancy on Eating Habits and Attitudes to Shape and Weight." *International Journal of Eating Disorders* 9 (1990): 153.

———. "Eating Habits and Eating Disorders During Pregnancy." *Psychosomatic Medicine* 54 (1992): 665.

"Families That Eat Together . . ." *Tufts University Health & Nutrition Letter,* October 1997, p. 2.

Fatourechi, V., et al. "Demystifying Autoimmune Thyroid Disease." *Symposium; Thyroid Disease* 107 (2000): 127.

Fink, G., et al. "Estrogen Control of Central Neurotransmission: Effect on Mood, Mental State and Memory." *Cellular and Molecular Neurobiology* 16 (1996): 325.

Fisher, H. 1999. *The First Sex.* New York: Random House.

Fisher, J. O., et al. "Parents' Restrictive Feeding Practices Are Associated with Young Girls' Negative Self-Evaluation of Eating." *Journal of the American Dietetic Association* 100 (2000): 1341.

Fitness: "Don't Sweat the Past."*Health,* March 2000, p. 24.

"Fitness Furniture." *UC Berkeley Wellness Letter,* September 1998, p. 8.

Flagler, S., et al. "Relationships Between Stated Feelings and Measures of Maternal Adjustment." *Journal of Obstetrics, Gynecological, and Neonatal Nursing* 19 (1990): 411.

Fly, A. D., et al. "Major Mineral Concentrations in Human Milk Do Not Change After Maximal Exercise Testing." *American Journal of Clinical Nutrition* 68 (1998): 345.

Foldspang, A., et al. "Parity as a Correlate of Adult Female Urinary Incontinence." *Journal of Epidemiological Community Health* 46 (1992): 595.

Forman, A., et al. "Size Matters: Reining in Out-of-Control Portions." *Environmental Nutrition* 23 (2000): 2.

Francis, C. C., et al. "Body Composition, Dietary Intake, and Energy Expenditure in Nonobese, Prepubertal Children of Obese and Nonobese Biological Mothers." *Journal of the American Dietetic Association* 99 (1999): 58.

Fraser, L. "Body Love, Body." *Glamour,* October 1998, p. 280.

Fynes, M., et al. "Effect of Second Vaginal Delivery on Anorectal Physiology and Faecal Continence: A Prospective Study." *Lancet* 354 (1999): 983.

"FYI: Women's Health Research News—Men Do Listen with Half a Brain." *Women's Health Advisor,* February 2001, p. 8.

Gjerdingen, D. K., et al. "Mothers' Experience with Household Roles and Social Support During the First Postpartum Year." *Women and Health* 21 (1994): 57.

"The Glycemic Index." *Harvard Women's Health Watch,* December 1999, p. 6.

Golay, A., et al. "Similar Weight Loss with Low-Energy Food Combining or Balanced Diets." *International Journal of Obesity and Related Metabolic Disorders* 24 (2000): 492.

Gold, P., et al. "Role of Glucose in Regulating the Brain and Cognition." *American Journal of Clinical Nutrition* 61 (1995): 987S.

Gore, A. 2000. *The Mother Trip.* Seattle: Seal Press.

Grace, J. T., et al. "Mothers' Self-Reports of Parenthood Across the First 6 Months Postpartum." *Research in Nursing and Health* 16 (1993): 431.

"Green Is for Girls." *Shape Presents Fit Pregnancy,* February/March 2001, p. 32.

Greene, G. W., et al. "Postpartum Weight Change: How Much of the Weight Gained in Pregnancy Will Be Lost After Delivery?" *Obstetrics and Gynecology* 71 (1988): 701.

Gruen, D. "Postpartum Depression: A Debilitating Yet Often Unassessed Problem." *Health and Social Work* 15 (1990): 261.

Hachey, D., et al. "Benefits and Risks of Modifying Maternal Fat Intake in Pregnancy and Lactation." *American Journal of Clinical Nutrition* 59 (1994): 454S.

Haddow, J. E., et al. "Maternal Thyroid Deficiency During Pregnancy and Subsequent Neuropsychological Development of the Child." *New England Journal of Medicine* 341(1999): 549.

Haffner, S. M., et al. "Leptin Concentrations in Women in the San Antonio Heart Study: Effect of Menopausal Status and Postmenopausal Hormone Replacement Therapy." *American Journal of Epidemiology* 146 (1997): 581.

Haines, P., et al. "Trends in Breakfast Consumption of US Adults Between 1965 and 1991." *Journal of the American Dietetic Association* (96) 1996: 464.

Hardie, L., et al. "Circulating Leptin in Women: A Longitudinal Study in the Menstrual Cycle and During Pregnancy." *Clinical Endocrinology* 47 (1997): 101.

Harris, H. E., et al. "The Impact of Pregnancy on the Long-Term Weight Gain of Primiparous Women in England." *International Journal of Obesity* 21 (1997): 747.

Hayslip, C. C., et al. "The Effects of Lactation on Bone Mineral Content in Healthy Postpartum Women." *Obstetrics and Gynecology* 73 (1989): 588.

Heitmann, L., et al. "Do We Eat Less Fat, or Just Report So?" *International Journal of Obesity and Related Metabolic Disorders* 24 (2000): 435.

Helland, I., et al. "Leptin Levels in Pregnant Women and Newborn Infants: Gender Differences and Reduction During Neonatal Periods." *Pediatrics* 101 (1998): 465.

Hickey, M., et al. "Gender-Dependent Effects of Exercise Training on Serum Leptin Levels in Humans." *American Journal of Physiology* 272 (1997): E562.

Hirsch, J., et al. "Methods for the Determination of Adipose Cell Size in Man and Animals." *Journal of Lipid Research* 9 (1968): 110.

Hochschild, A. R. 1997. *The Time Bind.* New York: Henry Holt.

Hogbin, M. B., et al. "Public Confusion over Food Portions and Servings." *The Journal of the American Dietetic Association* 99 (1999): 1209.

"Honey, I'm Stressed." *American Health,* May 1999, p. 18.

Horns, P., et al. "Pregnancy Outcomes Among Active and Sedentary Primiparous Women." *Journal of Obstetrics and Gynecology* 25 (1996): 49.

Horowitz, J. A., et al. "Mothers' Perceptions of Postpartum Stress and Satisfaction." *Journal of Obstetric, Gynecological, and Neonatal Nursing* 28 (1999): 595.

"Hostility and Fat." *Self,* August 1999, p. 110.

Howard, B. "Survey Says: *Shape* Readers on Body Image and Sex." *Shape,* September 1997, p. 118.

Huang, Z., et al. "Body Weight, Weight Change, and Risk for Hypertension in Women." *Annals of Internal Medicine* 128(1998): 81.

Hunter, G. R., et al. "Racial Differences in Energy Expenditure and Aerobic Fitness in Premenopausal Women." *American Journal of Clinical Nutrition* 71 (2000): 500.

Illingworth, P. J., et al. "Diminution in Energy Expenditure During Lactation." *British Medical Journal* 292 (1986): 437.

Iovine, V. 1995. *The Girlfriend's Guide to Pregnancy.* New York: Pocket.

———. 1997. *The Girlfriend's Guide to Surviving the First Year of Motherhood.* New York: Berkley.

———. 1999. *The Girlfriend's Guide to Toddlers.* New York: Berkley.

Jameson, M. "When Worlds Collide." *Shape Presents Fit Pregnancy,* February/March 2001, p. 42.

Janney, C. A., et al. "Lactation and Weight Retention." *American Journal of Clinical Nutrition* 66 (1997): 1116.

Jenkin, W., et al. "Psychological Effects of Weight Retained After Pregnancy." *Women and Health* 25 (1997): 89.

Joyce, T., et al. "An Update on New York City's Dramatic Increase in Low Birthweights." *American Journal of Public Health* 83 (1993): 109

Kahn, H. S., et al. "Relation of Birth Weight to Lean and Fat Thigh Tissue in Young Men." *International Journal of Obesity* 24 (2000): 667.

Kalkwarf, H. J., et al. "The Effect of Calcium Supplementation on Bone Density During Lactation and After Weaning." *New England Journal of Medicine* 337 (1997): 523.

———. "Effects of Calcium Supplementation and Lactation on Iron Status." *American Journal of Clinical Nutrition* 67 (1998): 1244.

Kanarek, R., et al. "Psychological Effects of Snacks and Altered Meal Frequency." *British Journal of Clinical Nutrition* 77 (1997): S105.

Kannan, S., et al. "Cultural Influences on Infant Feeding Beliefs of Mothers." *Journal of the American Dietetic Association* 99 (1999): 88.

Kant, A. K., et al. "A Prospective Study of Diet Quality and Mortality in Women." *Journal of the American Medical Association* 283 (2000): 2109.

Kayman, S., et al. "Maintenance and Relapse After Weight Loss in Women: Behavioral Aspects." *American Journal of Clinical Nutrition* 52 (1990): 800.

"Keep Weight Off by Adding Unsaturated Fats." *Environmental Nutrition,* July 2000, p. 8.

Keim, N., et al. "Weight Loss Is Greater with Consumption of Large Morning Meals and Fat-Free Mass Is Preserved with Large Evening Meals in Women on a Controlled Weight Reduction Regimen." *Journal of Nutrition* 127 (1997): 75.

Kelly, P., et al. "Unmetabolized Folic Acid in Serum: Acute Studies in Subjects Consuming Fortified Food and Supplements." *American Journal of Clinical Nutrition* 65 (1997): 1790.

Keppel, K. G., et al. "Pregnancy-Related Weight Gain and Retention: Implications of the 1990 Institute of Medicine Guidelines." *American Journal of Public Health* 83 (1993): 1100.

King, J., et al. "Energy Metabolism During Pregnancy: Influence of Maternal Energy Status." *American Journal of Clinical Nutrition* 59 (1994): 439S.

Kjos, S. L., et al. "Postpartum Care of the Women with Diabetes." *Clinical Obstetrics and Gynecology* 43 (2000): 75.

Klem, M. L., et al. "A Descriptive Study of Individuals Successful at Long-Term Maintenance of Substantial Weight Loss." *American Journal of Clinical Nutrition* 56 (1997): 239.

Knopp, R. H., et al. "Two Phases of Adipose Tissue Metabolism in Pregnancy: Maternal Adaptations for Fetal Growth." *Endocrinology* 92 (1973): 984.

Kopp-Hoolihan, L. E., et al. "Longitudinal Assessment of Energy Balance in Well-Nourished, Pregnant Women." *American Journal of Clinical Nutrition* 69 (1999): 697.

Krebs, N. F., et al. "Bone Mineral Density Changes During Lactation: Maternal, Dietary, and Biochemical Correlates." *American Journal of Clinical Nutrition* 65 (1997): 1738.

Kuijpens, J. L., et al. "Prediction of Postpartum Thyroid Dysfunction: Can It Be Improved?" *European Journal of Endocrinology* 139(1998): 36.

Laskas, J. M. "The Friendly Way to Beat Stress." *Health,* November/December 2000, p. 72.

Lazarus, J. H., et al. "Clinical Aspects of Recurrent Postpartum Thyroiditis." *British Journal of General Practice* 47 (1997): 305.

Lederman, S. A., et al. "Reproduction and Obesity: The Effect of Pregnancy Weight Gain on Later Obesity." *Obstetrics and Gynecology* 82 (1993): 148.

Lee, K. A., et al. "Parity and Sleep Patterns During and After Pregnancy." *Obstetrics and Gynecology* 95 (2000): 14.

Leermakers, E. A., et al. "Reducing Postpartum Weight Retention Through a Correspondence Intervention." *International Journal of Obesity and Related Metabolic Disorders* 22 (1998): 1103.

Leibowitz, S., et al. "Brain Neuropeptide Y: An Integrator of Endocrine, Metabolic and Behavioral Processes." *Brain Research Bulletin* 27 (1991): 333.

Levine, M. J. 1997. *I Wish I Were Thin, I Wish I Were Fat.* New York: Vanderbilt Press.

Li, V. "Sclerotherapy: Disappearing Act for Spider Veins." *Harvard Women's Health Watch,* July 2000, p. 4.

Lloyd, H., et al. "Acute Effects on Mood and Cognitive Performance of Breakfast Differing in Fat and Carbohydrate Content." *Appetite* 27 (1996): 151.

"Long Live Older Mothers." *Health,* December/November 1997, p. 17.

Lovelady, C. A., et al. "The Effect of Weight Loss in Overweight, Lactating Women on the Growth of Their Infants." *New England Journal of Medicine* 342 (2000): 449.

Lukas, M., et al. "Serum Cholesterol Concentration and Postpartum Depression." *British Medical Journal* 314 (1996): 143.

Maas, J. B. *Power Sleep.* New York: Villard, 1998.

MacArthur, C., et al. "Faecal Incontinence After Childbirth." *British Journal of Obstetrics and Gynecology* 104 (1997): 46.

Malabu, U. H., et al. "Increased Neuropeptide Y Concentrations in Specific Hypothalamic Regions of Lactating Rats: Possible Relationship to Hyperphagia and Adaptive Changes in Energy Balance." *Peptides* 15 (1994): 83.

Marchini, G., et al. "Plasma Leptin in Infants: Relations to Birth Weight and Weight Loss." *Pediatrics* 101 (1998): 429.

Marmonier, C., et al. "Metabolic and Behavioral Consequences of a Snack Consumed in a Satiety State." *American Journal of Clinical Nutrition* 70 (1999): 854.

Martell, L. K. "The Hospital and the Postpartum Experience: A Historical Analysis." *Journal of Obstetric, Gynecological, and Neonatal Nursing* 29 (2000): 65.

Maushart, S. 1999. *The Mask of Motherhood.* New York: Penguin.

McCrory, M. A., et al. "Randomized Trial of the Short-Term Effects of Dieting Compared with Dieting Plus Aerobic Exercise on Lactation Performance." *American Journal of Clinical Nutrition* 69 (1999): 959.

Melanson, K. J., et al. "Fat Oxidation in Response to Four Graded Energy Challenges in Younger and Older Women." *American Journal of Clinical Nutrition* 66 (1997): 860.

"The Mind-Baby Connection." *Health,* June 2000, p. 152.

Mitchell, T. "Cindy Crawford: Getting Back in Shape After the Baby." *USA Weekend,* April 21–23, 2000, p. 6.

Moran, C. F., et al. "What Do Women Want to Know After Childbirth?" *Birth* 24 (1997): 27.

"More Evidence for Exercise." *Harvard Women's Health Watch,* March 1999, p. 1.

Motil, K., et al. "Lean Body Mass of Well-Nourished Women Is Preserved During Lactation." *American Journal of Clinical Nutrition* 67 (1998): 292.

"Multiple Births for Older Women." *Harvard Women's Health Watch,* December 1999, p. 7.

Murphy, S. P., et al. "Changes in Energy Intakes During Pregnancy and Lactation in a National Sample of US Women." *American Journal of Public Health* 83 (1993): 1161.

Muscati, S. K., et al. "Timing of Weight Gain During Pregnancy: Promoting Fetal Growth and Minimizing Maternal Weight Retention." *International Journal of Obesity and Related Metabolic Disorders* 20 (1996): 526.

Neumark-Sztainer, D., et al. "Factors Influencing Food Choices of Adolescents: Findings from Focus-Group Discussions with Adolescents." *Journal of the American Dietetic Association* 99 (1999): 929.

"Obesity: Portions Out of Proportion." *Harvard Women's Health Watch,* August 2000, p. 1.

O'Dea, J. A., et al. "Male Adolescents Identify Their Weight Gain Practices, Reasons for Desired Weight Gain, and Sources of Weight Gain Information." *Journal of the American Dietetic Association* 101 (2001): 105.

Ohlin, A., et al. "Maternal Body Weight Development After Pregnancy." *International Journal of Obesity* 14 (1990): 159.

———."Trends in Eating Patterns, Physical Activity and Sociodemographic Factors in Relation to Postpartum Body Weight Development." *British Journal of Nutrition* 71 (1994): 457.

Oliwenstein, L., et al. "Caution: Working Mom." *Shape Presents Fit Pregnancy,* Fall 1999, p. 68.

Olsen L. C., et al. "Postpartum Weight Loss in a Nurse-Midwifery Practice." *Journal of Nurse-Midwifery* 31 (1986): 177.

"Overcome Genes: Get Fit." *Environmental Nutrition,* August 1999, p. 8.

Parham, E. S. "Promoting Body Size Acceptance in Weight Management Counseling." *Journal of the American Dietetic Association* 99 (1999): 920.

Parham, E. S., et al. "The Association of Pregnancy Weight Gain with the Mother's Postpartum Weight." *Journal of the American Dietetic Association* 90 (1990): 550.

Parker, J. D. "Postpartum Weight Change." *Clinical Obstetrics and Gynecology* 37 (1994): 528.

Parker, J. D., et al. "Differences in Postpartum Weight Retention Between Black and White Mothers." *Obstetrics and Gynecology* 81 (1993): 768.

Pinsker, B., et al. "Food Processing." *Shape,* February 2000, p. 54.

"Pleasure Principle." *UC Berkeley Wellness Letter,* September 1998, p. 8.

Pollitt, E., et al. "Does Breakfast Make a Difference in School?" *Journal of Dietetic Association* 95 (1995): 1134.

Porch, J. V., et al. "Aging, Physical Activity, Insulin-Like Growth Factor I, and Body Composition in Guatemalan Women." *American Journal of Clinical Nutrition* 66 (1997): 874.

Potter, S., et al. "Does Infant Feeding Method Influence Maternal Postpartum Weight Loss?" *Journal of the American Dietetic Association* 91 (1991):441.

Pugliese, M. T., et al. "Parental Health Beliefs as a Cause of Nonorganic Failure to Thrive." *Pediatrics* 80 (1987): 175.

Quandt, S. A. "Changes in Maternal Postpartum Adiposity and Infant Feeding Patterns." *American Journal of Physical Anthropology* 60 (1983): 455.

Raikkonen, K., et al. "Anger, Hostility, and Visceral Adipose Tissue in Healthy Postmenopausal Women." *Metabolism: Clinical and Experimental* 48 (1999): 1146.

Ravelli, A., et al. "Obesity at the Age of 50 in Men and Women Exposed to Famine Prenatally." *American Journal of Clinical Nutrition* 70 (1999): 811.

Rebro, S. M., et al. "The Effect of Keeping Food Records on Eating Patterns." *Journal of the American Dietetic Association* 98 (1998): 1163.

Reichman, J. 1998. *I'm Not in the Mood.* New York: Morrow.

Reynolds, J. L. "Post-Traumatic Stress Disorder After Childbirth: The Phenomenon of Traumatic Birth." *Canadian Medical Association Journal* 156 (1997): 831.

Rippe, J. M., et al. "The Role of Physical Activity in the Prevention and Management of Obesity." *Journal of the American Dietetic Association* 98 (1998): S31.

Ritchie, L. D., et al. "A Longitudinal Study of Calcium Homeostasis During Human Pregnancy and Lactation and After Resumption of Menses." *American Journal of Clinical Nutrition* 67 (1998): 693.

Roan, S. 2001. *Our Daughters' Health.* New York: Hyperion.

Rolls, B. J., et al. "Effects of Energy Density and Fat Content of Foods Affected Energy Intake in Lean and Obese Women." *American Journal of Clinical Nutrition* 69 (1999): 863.

Romon, M., et al. "Circadian Variation of Diet-Induced Thermogenesis." *American Journal of Clinical Nutrition* 57 (1993): 476.

Rookus, M. A., et al. "The Effect of Pregnancy on the Body Mass Index 9 Months Postpartum in 49 Women." *International Journal of Obesity* 11 (1987): 609.

Ross-Flanigan, N. "Kick Up Your Heels." *Health,* May 2000, p. 94.

Sadurskis, A., et al. "Energy Metabolism, Body Composition, and Milk Production in Healthy Swedish Women During Lactation." *American Journal of Clinical Nutrition* 48 (1998): 44.

Sampselle, C. M., et al. "Physical Activity and Postpartum Well-Being." *Journal of Obstetric, Gynecological, and Neonatal Nursing* 28 (1999):41.

Schauberger, C., et al. "Postpartum Weight Loss: Factors That Influence Weight Loss in the Puerperium." *Obestetrics and Gynecology* 79(1992): 424.

Schlundt, D., et al. "The Role of Breakfast in the Treatment of Obesity: A Randomized Clinical Trial." *American Journal of Clinical Nutrition* 55 (1992): 645.

Schoeller, D. A., et al. "How Much Physical Activity Is Needed to Minimize Weight Gain in Previously Obese Women?" *American Journal of Clinical Nutrition* 66 (1997): 551.

Scholl, T. O., et al. "Gestational Weight Gain, Pregnancy Outcome, and Postpartum Weight Retention." *Obstetrics and Gynecology* 86 (1995): 423.

Schwartz, M. W., et al. "The New Biology of Body Weight Regulation." *Journal of the American Dietetic Association* 97 (1997): 54.

"Self-Esteem Plummets After False Weight Feedback." *Eating Disorders Review,* November/December 1998, p. 5.

"Shape Up Your Body Image." *Tufts University Diet and Nutrition Letter,* May 1995, p. 8.

Sherwin, B., et al. "Hormones, Mood and Cognitive Functioning in Post-Menopausal Women. Estrogen and Mood." *Obstetrics and Gynecology* 87 (1996): 20S.

Sholomskas, D., et al. "Postpartum Onset of Panic Disorder; a Coincidental Event?" *Journal of Clinical Psychiatry* 54 (1993): 476.

Skinner, J. D., et al. "Transitions in Infant Feeding During the First Year of Life." *Journal of the American College of Nutrition* 16 (1997): 209.

———. "Fruit Juice Intake Is Not Related to Children's Growth." *Pediatrics* 103 (1999): 58.

Skoner, M. M., et al. "Factors Associated with Risk of Stress Urinary Incontinence in Women." *Nursing Research* 43 (1994): 301.

Smith, A., et al. "Effects of Breakfast and Caffeine on Cognitive Performance, Mood, and Cardiovascular Functioning." *Appetite* 22 (1994): 39.

Smith, R. W., et al. "Effect of Lactation on Lipolysis in Rat Adipose Tissue." *Lipids* 11 (1976): 418.

Snooks, S. J., et al. "Effect of Vaginal Delivery on the Pelvic Floor: A 5-Year Follow Up." *British Journal of Surgery* 77 (1990): 1358.

Spaaij, C. J. K., et al. "Effect of Lactation on Resting Metabolic Rate and on Diet- and Work-Induced Thermogenesis." *American Journal of Clinical Medicine* 59 (1994): 42.

Stacey, M. "Sex and Exercise." *Shape,* June 2000, p. 96.

———. "Your Mother, Your Body." *Shape,* November 2000, p. 76.

Stanner, S. A., et al. "Does Malnutrition in Uteri Determine Diabetes and Coronary Heart Disease in Adulthood? Results from the Leningrad Siege Study, A Cross Sectional Study." *British Medical Journal* 315 (1997): 1342.

Stein, A., et al. "Eating Habits and Attitudes in the Postpartum Period." *Psychosomatic Medicine* 58 (1996): 321.

Stein, T. P., et al. "Plasma Leptin Influences Gestational Weight Gain and Postpartum Weight Retention." *American Journal of Clinical Nutrition* 68 (1998): 1236.

Steingrimsdottir, L., et al. "Diet, Pregnancy, and Lactation: Effects on Adipose Tissue, Lipoprotein Lipase, and Fat Cell Size." *Metabolism* 29 (1980): 837.

Strang, V. R., et al. "Body Image Attitudes During Pregnancy and the Postpartum Period." *Journal of Obstetric, Gynecological, and Neonatal Nursing* 14 (1985): 332.

Strote, M. E. "Leg Up-Lifts, Don't Let Varicose Veins Get You Down." *Shape Presents Fit Pregnancy,* June/July 2000, p. 52.

———. "The Gain Game, All About Those Pregnancy Pounds." *Shape Presents Fit Pregnancy,* August/September 2000, p. 48.

Stubbs, R., et al. "Breakfasts High in Protein, Fat or Carbohydrates: Effects on Within-Day Appetite and Energy Balance." *European Journal of Clinical Nutrition* 50 (1996): 409.

Sullivan, D. "Growing Strong." *Shape Presents Fit Pregnancy,* Spring 1999, p. 71.

Sultan, A. H., et al. "Anal Sphincter Disruption During Vaginal Delivery." *New England Journal of Medicine* 329 (1993): 1905.

Swash, M., et al. "Faecal Incontinence: Childbirth Is Responsible for Most Cases." *British Medical Journal* 307 (1993): 37.

Thompson, J. L., et al. "Effects of Diet and Exercise on Energy and Expenditure in Postmenopausal Women." *American Journal of Clinical Nutrition* 66 (1997): 867.

Thorsdottir, I., et al. "Different Weight Gain in Women of Normal Weight Before Pregnancy: Postpartum Weight and Birth Weight." *Obstetrics and Gynecology* 92 (1998): 377.

Thys-Jacobs, S. "Calcium Carbonate and the Premenstrual Syndrome: Effects on Premenstrual and Menstrual Symptoms." *American Journal of Obstetrics and Gynecology* 179 (1998): 444.

———. "Micronutrients and the Premenstrual Syndrome: The Case for Calcium." *Journal of the American College of Nutrition* 19 (2000): 220.

"Time for Dinner!" *Health,* June 2000, p. 18.

"Trading Couches for Treadmills." *Health,* November/December 1999, p. 62.

Trayhurn, P., et al. "Regulation of Leptin Production: A Dominant Role for the Sympathetic Nervous System?" *Proceedings of the Nutrition Society* 57 (1998): 413.

Tribole, E. 1998. *Stealth Health.* New York: Viking.

Tucker, L., et al. "Dietary Fat and Body Fat: A Multivariate Study of 205 Adult Females." *American Journal Clinical Nutrition* 56 (1992): 616.

"Tune Out, Turn Off, Lose Weight." *UC Berkeley Wellness Letter,* February 2000, p. 8.

Tusa, S. "Baby Talk's Exclusive Mom vs. Mom Survey Report." *Babytalk,* September 2000, p. 40.

"Using Your Feet to Improve Your Brain Power." *Tufts University Health and Nutrition Letter,* September 1999, p. 3.

Van Raaij, J., et al. "Energy Cost of Lactation, and Energy Balances of Well-Nourished Dutch Lactating Women: Reappraisal of the Extra Energy Requirements of Lactation." *American Journal of Clinical Nutrition* 53 (1991): 612.

Viktrup, L., et al. "The Symptom of Stress Incontinence Caused by Pregnancy or Delivery in Primiparas." *Obstetrics and Gynecology* 79 (1992): 945.

"Vital Statistics." *Health,* June 2000, p. 24.

Waggoner, G., and D. Stumpf. 1999. *From Baby to Bikini.* New York: Warner.

Walker, L. "Predictors of Weight Gain at 6 and 18 Months After Childbirth: A Pilot Study." *Journal of Obstetrics and Gynecological Neonatal Nursing* 25 (1996): 39.

Walker, L. O., et al. "Mothering Behavior and Maternal Role Attainment During the Postpartum Period." *Nursing Research* 35 (1986): 352.

———. "Weight-Related Distress in the Early Months after Childbirth." *Western Journal of Nursing Research* 20 (1998): 30.

Walsh, J., et al. "Fitness for Life: How to Get the Most Out of Moving Your Body More." *Environmental Nutrition* 22 (1999): 1.

Ward, E. S. "Keeping Postmenopausal Pounds at Bay: Why Strength Training Is Key." *Environmental Nutrition* 24 (2001): 1.

Weeks, J., et al. "Gestational Diabetes: Does the Presence of Risk Factors Influence Perinatal Outcome?" *American Journal of Obsetrics and Gynecology* 171 (1994): 1003.

"Weight Cycling Is Linked to Gallstones." *Self,* August 1999, p. 110.

Weinberg, M. K., et al. "The Impact of Maternal Psychiatric Illness on Infant Development." *Journal of Clinical Psychiatry* 59 (1998): 53.

Weinsier, R. L., et al. "The Etiology of Obesity: Relative Contribution of Metabolic Factors, Diet, and Physical Activity." *American Journal of Medicine* 105 (1998): 145.

Welch, S. L., et al. "Life Events and the Onset of Bulimia Nervosa: A Controlled Study." *Psychological Medicine* 27 (1997): 515.

Weller, K. A. "Diagnosis and Management of Gestational Diabetes." *American Family Physician* 53 (1996): 2053.

Wells, A. S., et al. "Alterations in Mood After Changing to a Low-Fat Diet." *British Journal of Nutrition* 79 (1998): 23.

Whiffen, V., et al. "Infants of Postpartum Depressed Mothers: Temperament and Cognitive Status." *Journal of Abnormal Psychology* 98 (1989): 274.

Wilson, P. D., et al. "Obstetric Practice and the Prevalence of Urinary Incontinence Three Months After Delivery." *British Journal of Obstetrics and Gynecology* 103 (1996): 154.

Wisner, K., et al. "Anti-Depressant Treatment During Breast Feeding." *American Journal of Psychiatry* 154 (1997): 1174.

Index